HOW YOU GONNA GET TO HEAVEN IF YOU CAN'T TALK WITH JESUS

On Depathologizing Deafness

James Woodward

"Language and the Maintenance of Ethnic Boundaries in the Deaf Community" was first published in *Communication and Cognition* 1978, Vol. 11, No. 1. Reprinted with permission of Harry Markowicz and Werkgroep voor de studie van communiatieve and cognitieve processen.

"Some Sociolinguistic Problems in the Implementation of Bilingual Education for Deaf Students" was first published in the Proceedings of the *Second National Symposium on Sign Language Research and Teaching*, edited by Frank Caccamise and Doin Hicks, 1980, Silver Spring, MD.: National Association of the Deaf. Reprinted with permission of the National Association of the Deaf.

Parts of "Beliefs About and Attitudes Towards Deaf People and Sign Language on Providence Island" appeared in "Attitudes Towards Deaf People on Providence Island: A Preliminary Survey," *Sign Language Studies* 1977, No. 18.

T.J. PUBLISHERS, INC.
817 Silver Spring Avenue, 305D/Silver Spring,
Maryland 20910

Reprinted February 1989

Printed in the United States of America
ISBN #0-932666-15-9
Library of Congress Catalog No.: 82-51253

CONTENTS

Acknowledgements

Research on the article "How You Gonna Get to Heaven if You Can't Talk With Jesus: The Educational Establishment vs. the Deaf Community" was supported in part by NEH Research Grant RO-21418-75-196. Research on "Language and the Maintenance of Ethnic Boundaries in the Deaf Community" was supported in part by NSF Research Grant SOC 74-14724 and NEH Research Grant RO-21418-75-196. Research on "Beliefs About and Attitudes Toward Deaf People and Sign Language on Providence Island" was supported in part by NSF Research Grant BNS 76-80056. The findings and views presented in these papers do not necessarily represent the views of the granting agencies.

I would like to thank Lloyd Anderson, Susan De Santis, Carol Erting, Carolyn Ewoldt, and Robert Johnson for their comments and criticisms on "Some Sociolinguistic Problems in the Implementation of Bilingual Education for Deaf Students." In addition, I would like to thank Brenda Rawlings for supplying the general population percentages which I used in calculating my rough demographic figures for typical linguistic consultants for ASL. Finally, many thanks are due to Susan De Santis and Orva Henry for help in collecting data for "Beliefs About and Attitudes Toward Deaf People and Sign Language on Providence Island."

Introduction

The articles in this book were written between the years of 1975 and 1979. They relate to topics of the utmost concern for Deaf[1] people; however, they have not been widely disseminated in the fields related to deafness. "Language and the Maintenance of Ethnic Boundaries in the Deaf Community" was presented in 1975 at the Conference on Culture and Communication in Philadelphia. It was not published until 1978 in *Communication and Cognition*, a European journal not generally available in the U.S. "How You Gonna Get to Heaven if You Can't Talk With Jesus: The Educational Establishment vs. The Deaf Community" was presented in 1975 at the Annual Meeting of the Society for Applied Anthropology in Amsterdam. It has never been published until now.

The other two papers have been available to more people in the fields related to deafness, yet they too have been very limited in their distribution. "Some Sociolinguistic Problems in the Implementation of Bilingual Education for Deaf Students" was given at the Second National Symposium on Sign Language Research and Teaching in 1978 in San Diego and was published in the proceedings of the conference. However, only a comparatively small number of copies of the proceedings were published. Finally, a preliminary version of the last paper in this volume was published in *Sign Language Studies* in 1977. The *SLS* paper, however, only included research related to attitudes towards Deaf people on Providence Island and was only based on research from two villages on the island.

All four papers represent a development in research towards understanding Deaf society and culture in the U.S. and towards understanding why Hearing society in the U.S. has been so slow to give up the idea of Deaf people as pathological handicapped individuals. The four papers in this book view the U.S. Deaf community from anthropological and sociolinguistic perspectives. The papers attempt to describe Deaf people from

---

[1]The term "Deaf" in this paper refers to sociological deafness; the term "deaf" refers to audiological deafness. The term "Hearing" refers to those people who identify with oral language communities and their values; the term "hearing" means the ability to hear.

Even though Deaf people on Providence Island do not form a distinct sociological community from Hearing people, I have used the term "Deaf" to refer to them for these reasons: 1) Deaf on Providence Island use sign language and not an oral language, 2) the sign language greatly differs from the oral languages, and 3) on Providence neither Deaf people who sign nor Hearing people seek audiological solutions to deafness.

the point of view of Deaf cultural values. Thus differences between Deaf and Hearing people can be seen as cultural differences not as deviations from a Hearing norm.

The first two papers in this book focus on description of Deaf people as minority group members rather than as pathological individuals. "Language and the Maintenance of Ethnic Boundaries in the Deaf Community" discusses the Deaf community as an ethnic group in the U.S., specifically focusing on the role of language use as an internal and an external force in maintaining solidarity in the community. "How You Gonna Get to Heaven if You Can't Talk With Jesus: The Educational Establishment vs. The Deaf Community" relates how the U.S. Deaf community as an ethnic group has maintained linguistic and cultural identity despite strong oppression from the majority Hearing society.

The third paper in this volume relates to a logical application of the findings of the first two papers: bilingual education in ASL and English for Deaf students. Such bilingual education would be desirable for Deaf students; however, as the paper demonstrates, there are some large obstacles to overcome if one wants a successful program. Two of the biggest problems are that (1) the push for bilingual education must come from within the Deaf community to be successful, and (2) attitudes and behaviors of Hearing and Deaf must be positive toward Deaf people, ASL, English, and bilingual education before bilingual education can succeed. Ultimately, failure of a bilingual education program can be much more socially devastating than never beginning one.

The fourth article presents evidence from another society that demonstrates that Deaf people can be viewed in a relatively positive way by the majority of the Hearing members of the society and that a society can be structured so that Deaf and Hearing individuals can be integrated without sacrificing the integrity of either group as humans. This type of integration is in sharp contrast to American mainstreaming techniques which tend to be successful only to the extent that a Deaf child can become Hearing.

Finally, I have included a short summary and discussion entitled "On Depathologizing Deafness" which ties together the findings of the first four papers into a coherent philosophical framework for viewing Deaf people in the U.S.

Harry Markowicz and James Woodward

Language and the Maintenance of Ethnic Boundaries in the Deaf Community

In this paper we attempt to present first, a definition of the Deaf community, and second, a demonstration of the importance of language in maintaining the integrity of its social organization.

The extensive literature on deafness consists for the most part of psychological studies of deaf individuals. The purpose of these investigations is usually to compare the intelligence and performance of deaf people with those of hearing people. The results yielded by this type of research have been contradictory. Some studies conclude that the deaf are inferior to hearing people in some aspects of intelligence and performance (Myklebust 1960), while others find similar kinds of distribution in the two groups (Furth 1966).

The important point to note about these studies is that there is no recognition of the effects of the Deaf experience and of the Deaf subculture on the testing situation (Lunde 1960). The assumption is made by the testers that the only difference between the two groups is that one has the ability to hear, while the other does not. In other words, Deaf people are viewed as Hearing people, with the exception that they can't hear.

Some professionals who work with Deaf people have recently begun to recognize the existence of a Deaf minority, with a hierarchical social structure, its own culture and language (Lunde 1960, Vernon & Makowsky 1969, Meadow 1972). Members of the Deaf community include the profoundly deaf, the hard of hearing, the prelingually and the postlingually deaf, those who have intelligible speech as well as those who don't. The particular degree of hearing loss does not appear to be a criterion for membership. Rare instances of hearing members, for example some hearing children of Deaf parents, are also reported in the literature (Schlesinger 1972, Furth 1973). These ascriptions, however, may be questionable since they are made by Hearing researchers who are not themselves part of the community.

On the other hand, there are also both deaf and hard of hearing people who have no contact with the Deaf subculture. They do not identify with this minority and the members do not accept them into the community. A study (Padden & Markowicz 1976) was undertaken at Gallaudet College, a liberal arts college for hearing impaired students, involving the small minority of new students who had been previously enculturated in the Hearing community. Before entering Gallaudet College, this group of students had not interacted with other deaf people and they knew no sign language. The primary objective of that study was to follow the students' acculturation process and to note the kinds of cultural conflicts they encountered. After six months of submersion in the Deaf subculture, there was evidence that these students were still excluded from normal social interaction with fellow-students who are part of the Deaf community.

The most obvious barrier to participation in the Deaf community is linguistic. Gumperz (1975) expresses the intimate relationship between a community, its culture and its language: "Language is simultaneously a store or a repository of cultural knowledge, a symbol of social identity, and a medium of interaction." The primary language of the Deaf community is American Sign Language (ASL). Besides being its vernacular language, it serves also as the principal identifying characteristic of its members (Stokoe 1970, Woodward 1973a, Padden & Markowicz 1976).

The language situation in the Deaf community can best be described as a bilingual-diglossic continuum between ASL and English (Stokoe 1970, Woodward 1973a). Although the community is bilingual, most of its members do not have native competence in English. A small minority—some of the most highly educated prelingually deaf, the hard of hearing and the postlingually deaf—are proficient in English. Using reading tests as a measuring instrument, Furth (1966) found that only 12% of the deaf population demonstrates native-like competence in English

For the most part, prelingually deaf people are very limited in their ability to communicate orally. Their mechanically acquired speech is generally unintelligible to most people. They cannot easily depend on lipreading since this skill is difficult and presupposes a knowledge of the spoken language. Writing also depends on knowing English, but in addition, it is a tedious and slow mode of communication. By necessity interaction with Hearing people is limited.

In cross-cultural interaction "the majority culture expects to be addressed in its own language" (Weinreich 1968). However, professionals who work with Deaf people usually communicate through a system of coding English into a manual-visual channel by stringing out individual sign-words into English word order. The use of this system, called Manual English or Sign English, depends on knowing English. Since most Deaf people do not have complete control of this language, a continuum of language varieties has developed between ASL and English. These intermediate varieties have been shown to exhibit pidgin-like characteristics (Woodward 1973b, Woodward & Markowicz 1975). Variation along the ASL-to-English continuum is regular, rule-governed, and correlates with a hierachy of gross social variables. For example, people who are Deaf, people born of Deaf parents and people who learned signs before the age of six tend to use language varieties that more closely approach "pure" ASL, while people who are Hearing, people who have Hearing parents, and people who learned signs after the age of six tend to use language varieties less like "pure" ASL (Woodward 1973a).

Diglossia is another important aspect of the Deaf subculture. Signing that approaches English along the continuum serves as the "H" variety and tends to be used in formal interaction, such as in church, the classroom, lectures, and in conversation with outsiders. Signing that approaches ASL is more like the "L" variety in that it is used in less formal situations, such as intimate conversations. English is usually considered superior to ASL, while ASL is often regarded as ungrammatical or nonexistent. Sign language diglossia appears to be as stable as other diglossic situations.

Although extensive interaction may occur between members and outsiders, some sectors of activity are not normally included in cross-cultural relations. Extended communication involving an outsider does not occur in the ASL end of the continuum. If a Hearing person joins a conversation among Deaf people, code switching to English-like signing is the immediate response. In this way, Hearing people are prevented from learning ASL, and consequently, certain areas of the Deaf subculture remain inaccessible to non-members.

Marital patterns among Deaf people can be used to illustrate this point. Fay (1898) records an 85% rate of endogamous marriage. Rainer et al (1963) in a survey of New York, found that 95% marriages of women born deaf and 91% of marriages of women who became deaf at an early age were endogamous. Because the rate of postlingual deafness was much higher in the past due to disease, one can hypothesize that marital patterns have changed very little since the turn of the century and probably before that in the U.S. Deaf community. Woodward & Markowicz (1975) also point out that since not all women in the study by Rainer et al were necessarily members of the Deaf community, the percentage of marriages across the ethnic boundary is possibly reduced even further (Woodward 1975a).

Social deafness appears to vary from the behaviour of the so-called "Deaf-Deaf" to behavior that is characteristic of Hearing people. Cultural values manifested in the different degrees of Deaf behavior can be placed on a continuum similar to the language continuum described above.

While Deaf cultural values and behavior viewed objectively appear to rank on a continuum, members of the Deaf community dichotomize others as either members or non-members. These categorical choices are made by means of patterns of certain socially significant features. Thus, a boundary is drawn around the Deaf community and it can be viewed as an ethnic group with which members identify on the basis of a basic identity (Barth 1969). Ascription to the Deaf minority group seems primarily to be based on two criteria: (1) attendance in a residential school for the Deaf, and (2) communicative competence in ASL (Stokoe 1965).

The following demographic facts help explain why the socialization of deaf children takes different patterns. Less than ten percent of deaf children are born of Deaf parents. Their enculturation naturally takes place in the home. For the over 90% of deaf children who have Hearing parents, socialization depends largely on the schools they attend. About half of this group attend residential schools for the Deaf where they are socialized into the Deaf community by older Deaf children and their Deaf peers who have Deaf parents (Meadow 1972). Most young deaf children do not have any contact with Deaf adults.

The other half of the deaf children with Hearing parents attend special day schools for the deaf, or else they are integrated into regular schools. Generally, deaf children who do not have Deaf parents and who do not attend residential schools identify with the Hearing society in which they function with varying degrees of success. They do not normally interact with the members of the Deaf community. However, as noted above in reference to the Gallaudet study (Padden & Markowicz), some individuals become acculturated into the Deaf community later in life. Presumably, their new social identity in the Deaf community is more satisfying than the social role they acted out previously in the Hearing community.

Deaf children differ from their counterparts in other ethnic groups in two important ways. First, as stated above, enculturation into the Deaf subculture does not generally take place within the home. Deaf children of Hearing parents often feel alienated from their families. Contact with Deaf adults is extremely limited and it is not unusual for young Deaf children to imagine that they will grow up to be Hearing adults. This accounts for the important role played by Deaf children of Deaf parents and older Deaf children in the process of enculturation of young Deaf children.

The second difference from children of other ethnic groups is due to the fact that hearing impaired individuals are viewed by Hearing people as requiring the assistance of various specialists in the field of deafness, e.g. audiologists, speech therapists, teachers of the deaf, and counselors. Deaf people normally find themselves cast in the roles of pupil, client, patient, employee, while the individuals who play out the dominant roles of teacher, doctor, speech therapist, audiologist, counselor, and employer, are usually Hearing people. In these asymmetrical interactions, Deaf people are often treated as defective Hearing people, while their membership in a subculture is ignored or denigrated. Such encounters may have contributed to the formation of a "conquest" culture (Aceves 1974). Like certain other minority groups, the Deaf community generally does not participate in the control of its own institutions (Vernon & Makowsky 1969). In terms of its economic, political, and social relations to the Hearing society, the Deaf minority can be viewed as a colony.

Language varieties serve to delimit interaction within and between the Deaf and Hearing communities. Signing that approaches ASL is primarily used within the Deaf community for intimate interactions of members. Thus, the use of ASL-like signing serves to integrate Deaf people into the community and to assign to them social roles, while at the same time it excludes outsiders from intimate interactions with members.

Pidgin Sign English (PSE) serves as a linguistic and cultural buffer that allows for only minimal interaction between the Hearing and Deaf communities and then only for a limited group of Hearing and Deaf brokers (Woodward & Markowicz 1975). This group includes mostly college educated Deaf individuals—about 1–2% of the Deaf population, and Hearing professionals. PSE allows the transmission of information in a code native to neither Deaf nor Hearing individuals, but in a channel to which the Deaf person is clearly more attuned. Information useful to the community and its members can be obtained without sacrificing cultural integrity and group solidarity. There is little chance that Hearing people can actively introduce new and contradictory ideology into the community in a language other than ASL.

ASL serves as the primary criterion for identification of self and others as members of the Deaf subculture, and for the promotion of solidarity within the group. This social function is so important to the group that some community members may on occasion misidentify as a Deaf person a skilled Hearing signer whose signs approach ASL, especially in the extensive use of constructions like directionality in three dimensional space to represent agent-beneficiary relationships (Woodward 1975b). This is an extremely rare situation, since most Hearing signers are thwarted from learning ASL by the diglossic pressure that insures that Deaf signers will attempt to approach English when signing with an outsider. The misidentification is more likely to occur in locales where it is rare for Hearing people to sign at all, much less approach the language varieties that the Deaf community identifies with. Some foreign Deaf individuals, even of Deaf parents (Battison, personal communication), and some Deaf community members who acquired signs late in life, are also misidentified as Hearing people.

In rare situations where Hearing individuals manage to thwart the diglossic pressure, conflicts will arise as to what social role this person should have in relation to the Deaf community, since Hearing people are not supposed to sign like Deaf people. There seem to be two possible solutions to this conflict: a change in interaction patterns or continued interaction on the same (interpersonal) level. The most common way of handling this conflict is to reinforce the diglossic situation by code-switching to English-like signing. This may be viewed as a sanction for violation of expected cultural values and linguistic norms. This diglossic reinforcement effectively excludes the Hearing person from deep integrative or interpersonal interaction, since ASL, not English, is used by most Deaf people for these functions. This re-erection of cultural-linguistic boundaries should be viewed as part of the ethnic identification of insiders and outsiders in the Deaf community. By switching to PSE, the Deaf community member has properly relabeled the Hearing person as an outsider. Thus, the Hearing person is excluded from intimate personal interaction with the Deaf community, thereby contributing to the maintenance of its autonomy and integrity.

The other way of handling the conflict of identification is to continue interacting in ASL. This implies the possibility of future intimate interaction. The use of ASL means that the Hearing person is not rejected as an outsider, but is incorporated into the community structure. This incorporation, however, does not necessitate membership in the Deaf community but rather something like the status of friend to the community. Some skilled Hearing signers who can approach ASL may be able to continue for an indefinite time in the role of special friend.

The definition of the Deaf community proposed in this paper appears to account for both the assumed cultural continuum between the Deaf sub-culture and the majority culture, and the fact that cognitively there exists a dichotomy along ethnic lines. Illustrations of linguistic behavior in the Deaf community support the claim that its language situation plays an important role in the maintenance of an ethnic boundary. Thus, it contributes to the maintenance of the positive social identities and satisfying in-group interaction of its members.

References

Aceves, J.B. 1974. *Identity, Survival, and Change: Exploring Social/Cultural Anthropology*. Morrisontown: General Learning Press.

Bailey, C.J. 1973. *Variation and Language Theory*. Washington, D.C.: Center for Applied Linguistics.

Barth, F. (ed.). 1969. *Ethnic Groups and Boundaries*. Oslo, Norway: Johansen and Nielsen Boktrykkeri.

Fay, E.A. 1898. *Marriages of the Deaf in America*. Washington, D.C.: Volta Bureau, Quoted in Lunde 1960.

Furth, H. 1966. *Thinking Without Language*. New York: The Free Press.

Furth, H. 1973. *Deafness and Learning*. Belmont, California: Wadsworth Publishing Co.

Gumperz, J. 1974. Linguistic Anthropology in Society, *American Anthropologist* 76, 785–798.

Lunde, A. 1960. The Sociology of the Deaf. In *Sign Language Structure: An Outline of the Visual Communication Systems of the American Deaf*. William Stokoe, University of Buffalo, Occasional Paper 8.

Meadow, K. 1972. Sociolinguistics, Sign Language, and the Deaf Subculture. In O'Rourke, T.J. (ed.). *Psycholinguistics and Total Communication: The State of the Art*. Washington, D.C.: American Annals of the Deaf.

Myklebust, H.R. 1960. *The Psychology of Deafness*. New York: Grune & Stratton, Inc.

Padden, C. & H. Markowicz. 1976. Cultural Conflicts Between Hearing and Deaf Communities. In F.B. & A.B. Crammatte (eds.). *Proceedings of the VII World Congress of the World Federation of the Deaf*. Washington, D.C.: National Association of the Deaf.

Rainer, J.D., Altshuler, K.Z., and F.J. Kallmann (eds.). 1972. *Family and Mental Health Problems in a Deaf Population*. New York: State Psychiatric Institute, Columbia.

Schlesinger, H. 1972. Meaning and Enjoyment: Language Acquisition in Deaf Children. In O'Rourke, T.J. (ed.). *Psycholinguistics and Total Communication: The State of the Art*. Washington, D.C.: American Annals of the Deaf.

Stokoe, W. 1970. Sign Language Diglossia. *Studies in Linguistics* 21, 27–41.

Stokoe, W., D. Casterline, and C. Croneberg. 1965. *A Dictionary of American Sign Language*. Washington, D.C.: Gallaudet Press.

Vernon, M., and B. Makowsky. 1969. Deafness and Minority Group Dynamics. *The Deaf American* 21, 3–6.

Weinreich, U. 1968. *Languages in Contact*. The Hague: Mouton.

Woodward, J. 1973a. Some Observations on Sociolinguistic Variation and American Sign Language. *Kansas Journal of Sociology* 9, 191–199.

Woodward, J. 1973b. Some Characteristics of Pidgin Sign English. *Sign Language Studies* 3, 39–46.

Woodward, J. 1975a (1982). How You Gonna Get to Heaven if You Can't Talk With Jesus: The Educational Establishment vs. The Deaf Community. Presented at the annual meeting of the Society for Applied Anthropology, Amsterdam, March 1975. Published in this book.

Woodward, J. 1975b. Variation in American Sign Language Syntax: Agent-Beneficiary Directionality. In Fasold, R., and R. Shuy (eds.) *Analyzing Variation in Language*. Washington, D.C.: Georgetown University Press.

Woodward, J. 1976. Black Southern Signing. *Language in Society* 5, 211–218.

Woodward, J. and H. Markowicz. 1975 (1980). Some Handy New Ideas on Pidgins and Creoles: Pidgin Sign Languages. Presented at the International Conference on Pidgin and Creole Languages, Honolulu, Hawaii, January 1975. Published in Stokoe, W. (ed.), *Sign and Culture*. Silver Spring, Maryland: Linstok Press.

James Woodward

How You Gonna Get to Heaven if You Can't Talk With Jesus: The Educational Establishment vs. The Deaf Community

The U.S. Deaf Community offers us unique insights into the nature of how a minority group can maintain linguistic and cultural identity and integrity despite heavy majority oppression. The Deaf community has had to face many of the same linguistic and cultural pressures that various other minority groups in the U.S. have had to face: being viewed as inferior by the majority culture, schooling in an institutional setting, almost exclusive instruction under majority group teachers, discrimination in and exclusion from teacher training programs, forced instruction in the majority language, the prohibition of the minority language in the school, etc. However, the Deaf community has had three additional pressures which other groups have not had. (1) The Deaf community has had a more difficult time overcoming inferiority stereotyping by the majority culture than other minority groups, since Deaf people are viewed as a *medical* pathology. (2) In the Deaf community less than 10% of Deaf children have Deaf parents. Thus the majority of Deaf children belong to a different cultural group from their parents and must be enculturated into the minority group through means other than their parents. (3) The primary language of the Deaf community differs not only in code structure but in channel structure from the majority language. Because of this, language oppression has often been doubly severe for Deaf people.

Contrary to the Hearing ethnocentric view of Deaf people as isolated pathological individuals, Deaf people form a thriving community that is held together by such factors as self-identification as a Deaf community member (Padden and Markowicz 1976, Markowicz and Woodward 1975), language (Croneberg 1965, Meadow 1972, Woodward and Markowicz 1975), endogamous marital patterns, and numerous national, regional, and local organizations and social structures (Meadow 1972). Not all hearing impaired individuals belong to the Deaf community, in fact, audiometric deafness, the actual degree of hearing loss, often has very little to do with where a person relates in the Deaf community (Padden and Markowicz 1976).

Attitudinal Deafness (self identification as a member of the Deaf community and identification by other members as a member) appears to be the most basic factor determining membership in the Deaf community (Padden and Markowicz 1976, Markowicz and Woodward 1975). Attitudinal Deafness explains why some hard of hearing persons consider themselves Deaf, why some profoundly hearing impaired individuals claim to be hard of hearing or actually Hearing, and why some young hearing children of Deaf parents may refuse to speak for some time, even though they are quite capable of speaking.

Attitudinal Deafness also helps explain the high incidence of endogamous marital patterns among Deaf people. Fay (1898) records an 85% rate of endogamous marriage and Rainer and others (1963) in a survey of New York found that 95% of marriages of women born deaf and 91% of marriages of women who became deaf at an early age were endogamous. Remembering that the rate of postlingual deafness was much higher in the past due to disease, one can hypothesize that marital patterns have changed very little since the turn of the century and probably before that in the U.S. Deaf community. Also as Woodward and Markowicz (1975) point out, since not all women in the study by Rainer and others were necessarily members of the Deaf community, the percentages of marriages across the Deaf ethnic boundary is possibly reduced even further.

Attitudinal Deafness is always paralleled by appropriate language use. The language situation in the Deaf community can best be described as a bilingual-diglossic continuum between American Sign Language (ASL) and English (Stokoe 1970, Woodward 1973a). Intermediate varieties along this continuum have been shown to exhibit pidgin-like characteristics (Woodward 1973b, Woodward and Markowicz 1975). Variation along the ASL-to-English continuum is non-discrete, regular, rule-governed, and correlated with a hierarchy of gross social variables. For example, people who consider themselves Deaf, people who have Deaf parents, and people who learned signs before the age of six use language varieties that more closely approach "pure" ASL, while people who are Hearing, people who have Hearing parents, and people who learned signs after the age of six tend to use language varieties less like "pure" ASL. (Woodward 1973a).

Signing that approaches English along the continuum serves as H in the diglossic situation and tends to be used in formal conversations, such as in church, the classroom, lectures, and with Hearing people. Signing that approaches ASL tends to be used in smaller, less formal, more intimate conversations. Publicly, English is often considered superior to ASL, and ASL is often regarded as ungrammatical or non-existent. Signers generally feel that "grammatical" English should be used instead of ASL for teaching.

Much formal grammatical description has been done on English (in its spoken or written form), but only relatively recently has any research on ASL been done. Some signers feel that standardization is necessary, but sign language diglossia appears as stable as other diglossic situations. Deaf children generally learn ASL in the initial locus of enculturation into the Deaf community, normally the family for Deaf children of Deaf parents and the residential school for Deaf children of Hearing parents. Thus sign language diglossia in the U.S. shares the same sociolinguistic characteristics of other languages in diglossic situations (cf. Ferguson 1959, Fishman 1967).

However, no matter what amount of research in the Deaf community and comparative research in other communities can be presented at this time to demonstrate that Deaf people form a minority group with language varieties quite different from English, the Hearing-controlled educational establishment generally still rejects the idea of a Deaf minority group. If the Hearing educational establishment were to recognize the Deaf community as a legitimate minority group, they would soon be forced to admit they know nothing about the structure of the group and that Deaf people could probably help themselves a lot better than Hearing people can.

Such an admission, however, would be counter to the authoritarianism that Vernon, a psychologist, finds so prevalent in Deaf education. Vernon (1972; 15) states: "A deaf child or adult often symbolizes to the authoritarian the very weaknesses and defects he fears himself. Sign language makes the deafness visible whereas its repression 'hides' the defect. . . Obviously repressing sign language is the first step in the denial of the weakness which deafness symbolizes to the authoritarian. The repression is inevitably rationalized and intellectualized as it remains an unconscious or preconscious motive. . ." This authoritarianism has existed since the founding of deaf education and has often been manifested in self-proclaimed religious missionary zeal to save Deaf people, hence the title of this paper. Cochrane (1873) in an old discussion of how he viewed the way Deaf students influenced Hearing teachers sums up the religious ethnocentrism and authoritarianism quite well. From my personal experiences, similar attitudes all too prevalently appear in present-day teachers, although they are generally expressed with somewhat more restraint.

Cochrane feels that teaching Deaf students "does not build up the mind; nay, rather it has a tendency to pull down, to lower the standard of previously acquired literary attainments." (Cochrane 1873; 43). Nevertheless, "we are called to labor among those who have no concept of a God; who know nothing of the kind, loving, merciful Father of the universe; whose ears have been closed to the simplest facts of Bible history; whose minds are shrouded in ignorance as dark as that which has settled down upon any of the nations of the earth." (Cochrane 1873; 47). "The teacher's work is to lift the veil that shuts out the beauties and glories of heavenly Jerusalem. . .so that in time the pupil comes to understand the plan and need of redemption." (Cochrane 1873; 46). Not one to mince words, Cochrane at one point puts his case quite clearly by comparing his contacts with Deaf students to that of his colleagues involved in teaching Hearing children in public schools. "It is very different with the teachers in the public schools, academies, and higher institutions of learning. They are brought in contact with a higher order of intellect." (Cochrane 1873; 44).

These kinds of attitudes of Hearing superiority and Deaf inferiority have led to discrimination in the hiring of Deaf teachers (Moores 1972), especially for young Deaf children, since in almost all schools, whether manually or orally oriented, early education for Deaf children has often stressed speech at the expense of other subjects.

This discrimination has effectively cut off classroom models of Deaf adults for most students until high school age. Some students in residential schools have been lucky enough to have Deaf house parents in the dormitories. This helps, but such obvious job (and pay) discrimination does little to enhance self-concept of Deaf adults or children.

While such discrimination has occurred in other minority groups, it seems that discrimination against Deaf people resulting in language oppression is especially severe and probably will be harder to overcome because Hearing ideology and technology have labelled Deaf people as abnormal and patho-logical characterization is often merely transferred from the individual to the group. (cf. Markowicz and Woodward 1975).

The problem of discrimination in the policy of hiring minority teachers and the resultant language oppression is compounded by the family situation in the Deaf community.

As mentioned earlier, less than 10% of Deaf children have Deaf parents and are enculturated into the Deaf community in the home. The other more than 90% of Deaf children have Hearing parents and are normally encul-turated into the Deaf community in residential schools (Meadow 1972) or, more rarely, acculturated upon graduation from a Hearing high school (Lunde 1960, Meadow 1972), or upon entrance into Gallaudet College (Pad-den and Markowicz 1976). The majority of Deaf children of Hearing parents are enculturated into the Deaf community and its language through peer group Deaf children of Deaf parents or through slightly older Deaf children who have already been enculturated into the Deaf community. Thus most Deaf children have not received meaningful Deaf cultural input from teach-ers or family, since teachers and families are mostly Hearing. Authoritarian language oppression can very easily occur under these situations. As we have already seen, the schools have tended to repress sign language, espe-cially ASL, and input from Deaf adults; and, as we shall see, even those that permit sign language, discriminate against ASL, the language varieties that Deaf people normally identify with (Padden and Markowicz 1976,

Markowicz and Woodward 1975). Other minority group children often have a refuge in the home from such cultural and linguistic oppression. However, as we have seen, more than 90% of Deaf children who attended residential schools do not have parents who belong to the same minority group as they do. Thus Deaf children are much less protected from cultural and linguistic discrimination than children from other minority groups.

Now, let us look at some basic characteristics of this language oppression.

The major issue in language policy for Deaf education has been the oral-manual controversy. Unfortunately, the whole argument, which was started and continued by Hearing people (L'Epee and Heinicke) is based on the peripheral issue of channel (Woodward 1973c). (See Garnett (1968) for some of the earliest statements of this controversy.) Oralism has been advocated strongly since the 1880 International Conference of Teachers of the Deaf met in Milan and declared: "The Congress, considering the incontestable superiority of speech over signing in *restoring the deaf mute to society, and in giving him a more perfect knowledge of language,* declares that the oral method ought to be preferred to that of signs for the education of the deaf and dumb." (Italics added.) Needless to say, almost all delegates to the Conference were Hearing.

This statement, which has heavily influenced language policy in many schools for the Deaf, presumes that there is only one society and one language—the society of Hearing people and the oral language(s) that they use. That there are Deaf communities with their own languages was (and still is to many Hearing educators) an inconceivable violation of ethnocentric beliefs.

It should be pointed out that even the advocates of manualism are generally not purely manual but advocate a combined method of speech and signs that parallel English word order. This variety of signs may vary from the natural pidgin, Pidgin Sign English, that developed out of contact between ASL and English (Woodward 1973b, Woodward and Markowicz 1975) to the artificial sign systems designed to represent English (Bornstein 1973). While it was not necessarily openly stated in all manualist philosophy that signs should parallel English, it is next to impossible to speak English and sign ASL at the same time. One might just as well attempt speaking English and writing French at the same time.

Thus, until recently, there has never been any question that the language code in the classroom should approach English; the question has been through what channel could English be best represented and understood.

With such discrimination against Deaf people and their language in educational policy and with the majority of parents of Deaf children being Hearing, how has the Deaf community been able to maintain its own language? There seem to be three possible reasons for this.

One reason seems to be that the oppression which has confronted the Deaf community has greatly strengthened the ethnic bond that unites people who choose to identify with the Deaf community. Because most Deaf children have not normally had a refuge in the home from cultural oppression, they appear at a very young age to have formed very strong ethnic ties with their peer group to cope with outside threats against self-concept and identity. Some support for this idea comes from Vernon (1972; 13) who states that "prominent existing theories of schizophrenia would assume that the isolation resulting from congenital deafness would seriously enough impair affective functioning and object relations actually to cause schizophrenia. Deafness reproduces many of the key early experiences thought to be primary to this psychosis." However, comparatively speaking, Deaf people are as well adjusted as Hearing people. Early ethnic affiliation may be one of the chief strategies for coping with an essentially hostile environment that is not often overcome with much help from parents.

Deaf consultants have reported to me that they feel that they and other Deaf people who strongly identify with the Deaf community, if forced to interact with an unknown outsider, would rather communicate with a foreign Deaf person than with a Hearing American. This ethnosemantic classification of closer-to-more-distant outsiders helps support the idea of the great strength of ethnic identification with the Deaf community. The second possible reason for the thriving of ASL relates to the channel and code structure of ASL as compared with English. Because Deaf people have hearing impairments, they prefer to use languages channeled through a visual-manual modality rather than through an oral-aural modality. As Hymes (1964, 1968) has suggested and as research studies in American Sign Language (Bellugi and Fischer 1972) have shown, language codes are highly constrained by channel. Sign languages are not particularly dependent on linearity and concatenations of inflectional affixes as oral languages tend to be. Instead, sign inflections are most often represented on the surface through internal modifications of the sign. An example of this is Agent-Beneficiary directionality (Woodward 1975) in which the relationship between actor and receiver is represented by movement in three dimensional space by the verb sign, not by linear order of occurrence or by sequential affixing. Sign language phonologies also have a completely different phonetic base physiologically from oral language phonologies. Thus it is impossible to directly transmit oral language phonology in a sign language and vice-versa (Woodward and Markowicz 1975). It seems then that the visual-manual channel of ASL prohibits very great influence from English structure, which is constrained by a different channel.

Thirdly, the diglossic situation in the Deaf community serves as a way of maintaining linguistic and cultural integrity. ASL is preserved since ASL and Pidgin Sign English have completely separate social functions. ASL is used for intimate interaction among members of the Deaf community. Pidgin Sign English is used in classroom situations and in conversations with Hearing people. With these separate functions, there is less likelihood of encroachments from English and a greater possibility of linguistic autonomy within the community. Also because the diglossic situation ensures that Deaf people switch to signing that approaches English around a Hearing person, most Hearing people are effectively barred from learning ASL and thus from actively influencing it. Furthermore, because Pidgin Sign English is a pidgin, it allows for satisfaction of basic communicative but not of integrative or expressive communication needs of members of the Deaf community. Thus, Pidgin Sign English "allows the transmission of information in a code native to neither Deaf nor Hearing individuals, but in a channel to which the Deaf person is clearly more attuned. Information useful to the community and its members can be obtained without sacrificing cultural integrity and group solidarity. There is little chance that Hearing people can actively introduce new and contradictory ideology into the community in a language other than ASL." (Markowicz and Woodward 1975: 9).

The Deaf community's preservation of linguistic and cultural traditions in the face of strong oppression exemplifies the ability of people to adapt for survival. In addition to pressures faced by other minority groups, the Deaf person has been viewed as a medical pathology, has undergone oppression of linguistic channel and code, and has not often had refuge in the home from sociolinguistic discrimination. The equalizing forces that have allowed the Deaf community to maintain minority language in spite of majority pressure are both social and linguistic. The strengthening of the ethnic bond is a social phenomenon, but it is tied to language, since one of the primary criteria for recognition of Deaf community members is the use of American Sign Language. The manual-visual channel preferred by Deaf individuals does not allow for easy transfer of information from a code transmitted in an oral-aural channel, e.g. English. Finally, the diglossic situation and the pidgin-like nature of Pidgin Sign English provide sociolinguistic buffers that permit American Sign Language to flourish with comparatively little outside influence.

References

Bellugi, U. and S. Fischer. 1972. A Comparison of Sign Language and Spoken Language. *Cognition* 1–2/3, 173–200.

Bornstein, H. 1973. A Description of Some Current Sign Systems Designed to Represent English. *American Annals of the Deaf* 18:1, 41–463.

Cochrane, M.A. 1873. What Influence has Teaching the Deaf and Dumb Upon the Teacher Himself? *American Annals of the Deaf* 18:1 41–49.

Croneberg, C. 1965. The Linguistic Community. In William Stokoe, Dorothy Casterline, and Carl Croneberg, *A Dictionary of American Sign Language.* Washington, D.C.: Gallaudet College Press, 297–312.

Fay, E.A. 1898. *Marriages of the Deaf in America.* Washington, D.C.: Volta Bureau.

Ferguson, C. 1959. Diglossia Word 15, 325–340.

Fishman, J. 1967. Bilingualism With and Without Diglossia; Diglossia With and Without Bilingualism. *Journal of Social Issues* 23:2, 29–38.

Gallaudet, E.M. 1873. "Deaf-Mute" Conventions, Associations, and Newspapers. *American Annals of the Deaf* 18:2, 200–206.

Garnett, C. 1968. *The Exchange of Letters Between Samuel Heinicke and Abbe Charles Michel De L'Epee.* New York: Vantage Press.

Hymes, Dell. 1964. Towards Ethnographies of Communication. In John Gumperz and Dell Hymes, editors, *The Ethnography of Communication. American Anthropologist* 66:6, 1–34.

_____. 1968. The Ethnography of Speaking. In Joshua Fishman, editor, *Readings in the Sociology of Language.* Mouton: The Hague, 99–138.

Lunde, A. 1960. The Sociology of the Deaf. In William Stokoe, *Sign Language Structure: An Outline of the Visual Communication Systems of the American Deaf. Studies in Linguistics,* Occasional Paper 8. 21–28.

Markowicz, H. and J. Woodward. 1975 (1978, 1982). Language and the Maintenance of Ethnic Boundaries in the Deaf Community. A paper presented at the conference on Culture and Communication, Philadelphia, March, 1975. Published in *Communication and Cognition* and in this book.

Meadow, K. 1972. Sociolinguistics, Sign Language, and the Deaf Subculture. In T.J. O'Rourke, editor, *Psycholinguistics and Total Communication: The State of the Art.* Washington, D.C.: The American Annals of the Deaf. 19–33.

Moores, D. 1972. Communication: Some Unanswered Questions and Some Unquestioned Answers. In T.J. O'Rourke, editor, *Psycholinguistics and Total Communication: The State of the Art.* Washington, D.C.: The American Annals of the Deaf. 1–10.

Padden, C. and H. Markowicz. 1976. Cultural Conflicts Between Hearing and Deaf Communities. In F.B. and A.B. Crammatte (eds.), *Proceedings of the VII World Congress of the World Federation of the Deaf.* Washington, D.C.: National Association of the Deaf.

Rainer, J.D., K.Z. Altshuler, and F.J. Kallmann, editors, 1963. *Family and Mental Health Problems in a Deaf Population.* New York: N.Y. State Psychiatric Institute, Columbia.

Stokoe, W. 1970. Sign Language Diglossia. *Studies in Linguistics* 21, 27–41.

Vernon M. 1972. Nonlinguistic Aspects of Sign Language, Human Feelings and Thought Process. In T.J. O'Rourke, editor, *Psycholinguistics and Total Communication: The State of the Art.* Washington, D.C.: The American Annals of the Deaf. 11–18.

Woodward, J. 1973a. Some Observations on Sociolinguistic Variation and American Sign Language. *Kansas Journal of Sociology* 9:2, 191–200.

_____. 1973b. Some Characteristics of Pidgin Sign English. *Sign Language Studies* 3, 39–46.

_____. 1973c. Deaf Awareness. *Sign Language Studies* 3, 57–59.

_____. 1975. Variation in American Sign Language Syntax: Agent-Beneficiary Directionality. In Ralph Fasold and Roger Shuy, editors, *Analyzing Variation in Language.* Washington, D.C. Georgetown University Press. 303–311.

Woodward, J. and H. Markowicz. 1975 (1980). Some Handy New Ideas on Pidgins and Creoles: Pidgin Sign Languages. A paper presented at the 1975 International Conference on Pidgin and Creole Languages, Honolulu, January, 1975. Published in Stokoe, W. (ed.), *Sign and Culture.* Silver Spring, MD: Linstok Press.

James Woodward

Some Sociolinguistic Problems in the Implementation of Bilingual Education For Deaf Students

Introduction

Bilingual education for any social group is not merely a linguistic problem. It is primarily a sociolinguistic problem. That is, the comparative grammatical structures of the languages in the school situation are of minor importance. What is important is the interaction of language and sociological issues; for example, a knowledge of language attitudes is more important than a knowledge of the linguistic structures of the two languages in determining the probable success or failure of bilingual education for a certain group. John and Horner (1971) point out: "If research on bilingualism is to be effective, it must go beyond the narrow confines of purely linguistic and psychological studies" (p. 106). "In other words," as Paulston (1974) states, "the most valid implication language planning can draw from language learning theory lies exactly in those factors the theory cannot account for. The limited answer we can draw on from language learning theory indicates the necessity of adopting a sociolinguistic and anthropological framework for examining solutions to sociolinguistic problems" (p. 27). In addition to sociolinguistic attitudes, a knowledge of the ethnography of communication (Hymes, 1964) of a given situation or the sociolinguistic influences of participants, topic, setting, channel, message form and their interrelationships on language preference, and use, is required. Even if we know a lot about the grammar of both languages, this knowledge in itself is not sufficient for establishing a bilingual education program.

Applying this general information about bilingualism to the sign language situation in the U.S., we can see that the chief problems to establishing bilingual education programs for Deaf students lie *not* in our comparative lack of knowledge of the structure of ASL, but in the language attitudes of Hearing and Deaf individuals and in the sociolinguistic parameters that influence the use of ASL.

This paper will attempt to point out *some,* not all, of the sociolinguistic problems that will interfere with the establishment of bilingual education programs for Deaf individuals. We will specifically look at (1) the widespread negative attitudes towards deaf people, towards ASL and towards the idea of bilingual education for Deaf students; (2) how diglossia can function as a specific barrier to the establishment of bilingual education for the Deaf; (3) the types of bilingualism that already occur in the Deaf community and problems this creates for bilingual education; and (4) language variation in ASL and the problem of acceptance of students' language varieties. These seem to be the most immediately crucial problems facing bilingual education for Deaf people. However, be aware that there are many other linguistic and sociolinguistic problems that will not be discussed in this paper.

While bilingual education is a very desirable alternative in the education of Deaf students, no one should attempt to start a bilingual education program for the Deaf unless (1) core members of the Deaf community (not just hearing impaired individuals) share *equally* in the control, administration, and teaching in any bilingual program or tract for Deaf individuals and (2) the bilingual program allows the free use of American Sign Language in and for itself (not merely for teaching English).

If the attitudinal and other sociolinguistic problems mentioned in this paper are not understood and/or unless the conditions I mentioned above are included in the proposed bilingual program, then it will probably be worse to attempt bilingual education than to merely leave the sociolinguistic situation alone. If the suggestions are not taken seriously, bilingual education will face the same problem that so-called "total communication" faces today. This problem requires some explanation. A number of schools are claiming that they use "total communication" (what they really mean most of the time is simultaneous communication), when in fact the majority of teachers can't sign their way out of a paper bag. Worse, the majority of teachers can't understand their students' signing. The "new" trend in "total communication" has every chance of failing, not because it is necessarily a bad idea (if any given definition of total communication considers ASL on a par with English, total communication and bilingual education are probably identical), but because *no one is doing what they say they are doing.* That is, there has been no real change in the education system. Teachers who could not and did not sign because of oral programs are too often still not able and/or willing to sign under so-called "total communication" programs. Changing the name of a program from oral to total communication does not change the program. The same problems exist under any name, if no substantial changes are made in content. One of the greatest problems of Deaf education is that everyone tries to jump on the latest bandwagon approach without being prepared and often without any real push to make substantive changes. People say "total communication" is the answer. Such an approach is simplistic. There is no one answer, no cure-all, no panacea. We don't even know all of the questions we should be asking. There are already many complex answers to the questions we have asked. How can there be just one answer?

The one answer cure-all bandwagon approach will not work for "total communication" and it will not work for bilingual education. Programs must be carefully assessed for feasibility and carefully designed if they have a chance of success. If teachers do not actually begin to sign in total communication programs and if bilingual education programs are not set up carefully, they will probably fail. The result could very well be a very swift and drastic reactionary shift to oralism within fifty years and possibly less time.

The reason for this should be clear. If there are no substantial changes in programs, research evaluations will show no significant improvement with these programs. Programs that were not "total communication" and that had problems because teachers couldn't sign, will still have the same problems if they call themselves "total communication" and the teachers still can't sign. Programs that call themselves bilingual that are not really bilingual will damage evaluations of good bilingual programs. Total communication and bilingual programs are more difficult to set up than strict oral programs, because they require much more training of personnel than oral programs. I don't think we should be so naive as to expect that people will be willing to support programs that require more effort and money and yet do not show significantly different affects. If a school does not have the resources to establish a bilingual education program, it should not. However, even if a school cannot establish a bilingual program at the present time, there are still positive changes that can be made. (We will discuss some of these positive changes in the conclusion). Zappert and Cruz (1977) point out that even if bilingual education shows a non-significant research finding, that this can still be interpreted as a positive effect since "students in bilingual classes have the added advantage of learning a second language and culture without impeding their education progress" (p. 39). However, I am somewhat skeptical that most business-minded legislatures or funding agencies are really satisfied with a result that is more than likely too intangible for them.

The Problems of Negative Attitudes

Negative attitudes towards ASL have been widespread for many years. It is not uncommon in diglossic situations (Ferguson 1959, Stokoe 1970) for some language varieties, generally the conversational varieties, to be looked down upon by outsiders and some insiders.

Linguists who study American Sign Language have frequently remarked that the mainstream attitude in both Hearing and Deaf communities has been that American Sign Language has no grammar or is poor or broken language (see for example Markowicz, 1972). Battison and Jordan (1976) point out the problem quite well:

> Others believe that sign languages have no grammar, no 'proper' ways of expressing things, but merely 'throw together' gestures and pan-tomimic actions; or they believe that sign languages abridge and corrupt correct spoken language grammar. These myths have been treated in recent years by other researchers, who find that the formal structures and communicative functions of sign languages used by deaf people are comparable to those of spoken languages used by hearing people (Stokoe, 1960, 1970; Woodward, 1973; Battison, 1974; Bellugi and Klima, 1975; Baker 1975; Frishberg, 1975; Klima and Bellugi, 1975; Liddell, 1975; Padden and Markowicz, 1975; Stokoe and Battison, 1975). (p. 53).

But, empirical research usually has little effect on attitudes. Witness the following classical attitudes from George Johnston, "Who has been deaf since the age of five and is presently only a dissertation short of a doctorate in special education administration, (and who) is director of Project PALS, a federally-funded statewide project designed to provide alternate language skills for Deaf students" (Marose, 1977).

> What Belugi (sic) in California and other people are calling American Sign Language or Ameslan, or As lazy and brief as they like to get ASL is actually Deaf English. DEAF ENGLISH is the typical errors (from improper or insufficient or unclear exposure) to English. It is a choice of words, a sub-culture style, omissions and additions, etc.
> . . .
> Give an English paragraph to 100 deaf people and ask them to sign it in American Sign Language. You will find them all different—no syntax. Only some common habits will be noticed . . . Then I argue, "What is a syntax?" How can you call American Sign Language something with a syntax when syntax involves sentence structure. Ridiculous, it is just Broken English or DEAF ENGLISH. (Johnston 1977, p. 22).

With such inaccurate information and negative attitudes towards ASL, (as manifested in the quote above), it is no wonder why there are negative attitudes towards bilingual education for Deaf students. To give you some examples of what I mean by negative attitudes, I would first like to share just *a few* of the negative experiences I have had when I have advocated bilingual education for Deaf people.

My first experience with talking about bilingual education to educators of the Deaf came in the summers of 1971 and 1972 at the jointly sponsored NAD/BEH institutes on psycholinguistics and total communication. After my discussion of the desirability of bilingual education for Deaf children, it was obvious that many of the students did not understand what I had said. These students believed that I was advocating only teaching ASL and that I was not advocating teaching English. I had never said that English should not be taught. All I had said was that ASL had a place in Deaf education. These students showed a naive attitude toward language learning. The naive view of bilingual education assumes that children in a bilingual program will learn less of the majority language (English) than if they were in a monolingual English program, since the children would be exposed to less English. However, research findings contradict this naive view. Lambert (1978), one of the foremost researchers in bilingual education points out: "the research of Padilla and Long (1969); (see also Long and Padilla, 1970) indicates that Spanish-American children and adolescents can learn English better and adjust more comfortably to America if their linguistic and cultural ties with the Spanish-speaking world are kept alive and active from infancy on." (p. 27). Lambert in the same article goes on to demonstrate that experiments carried out by his group in the northern regions of Maine showed a positive affect of English language learning when part of the education was conducted in French, the native language of a large number of families in that part of the U.S. When children were permitted to have "about a third of the elementary curriculum in French" (Lambert, 1978), (p. 30), they "clearly out-performed those French-speaking (students) in the control (monolingual in English) schools on various aspects of *English* language skills and on academic content, such as math." (Lambert, 1978) (p. 30). After five years of schooling the bilingually instructed French-speaking children performed not only better in French but also *in English,* as stated above, as compared with French-speaking children who had received all of their education in English.

My first experience with talking directly to teachers and administrators on their own turf, that is, at their own school came early in the Spring of 1973 when I had just started seriously to work on regional and ethnic variation in ASL. I spoke at one of the schools for the Deaf in the area where I was doing research explaining that I was studying regional and ethnic variation in ASL so that local schools might be best able to make use of their students' language in a bilingual program of ASL and English. After I finished, there was little response except from the Principal who said: "These students will learn English even if it is over my dead body." Another obvious misunderstanding of what bilingual education means.

Well, it so happens that after two years of off-and-on research around that area, I was invited to teach a course in that area, since several of the teachers apparently wanted a course in linguistics. I asked exactly what the teachers wanted to know, planned the course to cover exactly what they had requested, and arrived to find that only one teacher from the school was registered for the course. (Other teachers came from several other schools). Since that teacher left very soon to go back to graduate school, I doubt if very many ideas from the course reached the other teachers and especially the students in the school.

Moreover, during the course, I learned that the school was planning on revising its language (here read English only) curriculum. I talked with several administrators and teachers about the possibility of my consulting free of charge with only my transportation and living expenses paid for. I was never asked. The consultant they finally hired was an educator, not a linguist, who has not to my knowledge published any papers of the structure of any variety of sign language. While I do not have written proof that all of the above happened, I do have written proof in another situation, where a different school wanted information on "Signs for Sexual Behavior" (Woodward, 1979). Since the telephone call contained so many negative attitudes towards these signs in ASL, I even offered to pay my way including hotel expenses for a chance to discuss the need for selecting signs that were already in use by the local Deaf community. I was told by the administrator who called me that s/he did not have authority to invite me to come, but that s/he would check with the administrator who did have the authority and get back to me. I was never contacted again.

Skipping a number of other similar situations, we come to the Fall of 1977. Then I talked with the administrator who had told me in 1973 that the students would learn English over his dead body. Now he said they were using this brand new method of one sign for every English word. After spending about a half hour trying to explain to him that this idea was not new but certainly had a lot of problems, I suddenly realized that it did not make a hell of a lot of difference what I said or what research I showed such people. If people have such strong negative attitudes, they really were not interested in paying attention, no matter how open they said they were.

In addition to my anecdotal evidence, there are two other situations that should be briefly discussed.

The National Center for Law and the Deaf at Gallaudet College petitioned the Department of Health, Education, and Welfare, Office of Education, Office of General Counsel for Elementary and Secondary Schools, for a ruling that sign language be considered a language for use in bilingual study projects under the Bilingual Education Act, Title VII of the Elementary and Secondary Education Act of 1965, (20 USC 880b). The Law Center offered supporting sociolinguistic evidence for the use of ASL by Deaf persons and linguistic evidence that ASL was a language separate from English. While the government office has taken over a year and still has issued no written response, unofficial reports from telephone conversations indicate that sign language has been turned down as a language to be funded under the Bilingual Education Act.

Prickett and Hunt (1977) surveyed 122 experts in the field of education of the deaf who will be in a decision-making role during the next ten years. On a scale from 1 (most desirable) to 48 (least desirable) "Acceptance of bilingualism—sign and English" ranked 42.5 out of 48 as a 'high desirability' item, a very low rating. In addition "acceptance of bilingualism—sign and English" did not even make the list of 'high likelihood items'. Without acceptance of bilingualism, there can be no bilingual education. As Paulston (1974) points out: "Subject matter instruction in the native tongue (alone) is not sufficient to bring about significant results" (in bilingual education) . . . "In bilingual programs where mother-tongue instruction seems to be the causal factor in school achievement, it is presumably not for linguistic reasons but for the changed *attitudes* on the part of students and teachers which go with recognizing the status of the home language, normally stigmatized, as worthy of school use. Mother tongue instruction of minority languages usually implies that the teacher comes from the same reference group, from the same minority culture, and that by willingly speaking the native tongue, he demonstrates an acceptance of that culture." (p. 24). Paulston here is echoing the earlier comprehensive study of bilingual research by Diebold, (1966), who found that bilingualism had negative affects only when one of the languages was looked down upon.

We have tried to demonstrate that negative attitudes towards ASL and bilingual education in the Deaf community are widespread and long-standing. Attitudes are very stable and extremely difficult to change. We should expect that negative attitudes will continue as long as the majority culture's myth of the melting pot is maintained. (Later, when we discuss the large number of minority groups in this country which still use their own languages, it will become obvious why the belief in the melting pot is a myth.)

To understand these negative attitudes, we need to look at research on bilingualism in general as well as our society's beliefs about bilingualism.

Bilingualism and Bilingual Education

It should be pointed out that research related to the advantages and disadvantages of bilingualism and bilingual education can appear to be quite contradictory. The main reason for this is the poor research design of many studies, especially earlier studies of bilingualism. Zappert and Cruz (1977) in *Bilingual Education: An Appraisal of Empirical Research* had to reject 105 out of 108 project evaluations and 67 out of 76 research studies "due to one or more serious methodological weaknesses." (p. 39). They include a comprehensive list of all the research studies and project evaluations that they reviewed with the reasons why they excluded the studies.

There have been studies on such areas as the relationship of bilingualism and intelligence, and bilingualism and character formation, among others. Generally older studies are less well designed and tend to show more negative results than more experimental modern studies. Some earlier studies such as Saer (1923) on Welsh and English bilinguals tend to show negative effects of bilingualism on intelligence. Other studies such as the South African Bilingual Survey (Malherbe, 1934) showed that children bilingual in English and Afrikaans were more intelligent than monolingual children. Both of these studies, however, did not consider socio-economic status as a variable. Recently more sociologically sophisticated research by Peal and Lambert (1962) shows "that when groups of bilingual and monolingual children (French and English) are matched for the socio-economic status of their parents the bilinguals perform at least as well on I.Q. tests and have the added advantage of knowing a second language." (Saville and Troike, 1970, p. 1). Research on character formation shows equally disparate results. In a rather speculative study, Gali (1928) "has suggested that bilingual persons may be morally depraved because they do not receive effective religious instruction in their mother tongue in childhood (Weinreich, 1968, p. 119). Fishman (1951), however, has experimentally demonstrated that there was no significant relationship between the degree of bilingualism, friendship, and leisure habits of young children who used Yiddish and English. In a review of the literature on bilingualism, Diebold (1966) showed that negative effects of early bilingualism occurred only when one of the languages was looked down upon. More recently Zappert and Cruz (1977) have demonstrated:

> Most of the studies which remain show a significant positive effect, or a non-significant effect on student performance. Of the 77 findings reported here, only one (1%) was negative, 38 (58%) were positive, and 27 (41%) were neutral.
>
> As mentioned earlier, a non-significant effect is not a negative finding with respect to bilingual education. A non-significant effect, that students in bilingual education classes are learning at the same rate as students in monolingual classes, demonstrates the fact that learning in two languages does not interfere with a student's academic and cognitive performance. Students in bilingual classrooms have the added advantage of learning a second language and culture without impeding their educational progress. Under these circumstances, a non-significant finding can be interpreted as a positive effect of bilingual education. . . .
>
> Thus, the research demonstrates that bilingual education and bilingualism improves, or does not impede, oral language development, reading and writing abilities, mathematics and social studies achievement, cognitive functioning and self image. (p. 39).

Negative attitudes towards bilingualism are generally due to ethnocentrism and a lack of exposure to a variety of cultural situations. U.S. citizens on the whole have been remarkably intolerant of minority group languages. Apparently most Americans are unaware that bilingualism and bilingual education are worldwide phenomena that are considered normal in most of Europe, Asia, Africa, and South America. In these areas, bilingualism is seen as something that happens normally through social interaction, not something that is to be striven for or avoided. Macnamara (1967) in a discussion of some of the more *obvious* examples of bilingualism in Europe includes:

> The Catalans, Basques and Galicians in Spain; the Bretons and Provencials in France; the Welsh and Scots in the United Kingdom; the Flemings and Waloons in Belgium; the Romanish in Switzerland; the Valoise, Piedmonteso, Germans in Italy; the Frisians in Holland; the Laps throughout Scandinavia; the Italians, Hungarians, Slovenes, Croatians, Albanians and Macedonians in Yugoslavia; the Germans, Poles, and Slovaks in Czechoslovakia; the Germans and Ukrainians in Poland; the Hungarians in Rumania; the Macedonians in Bulgaria; the Turks in Cyprus; the Greeks in Turkey; the Finns, Estonians, Latvians, Lithuanians, White Russians, Ukrainians, Germans, Jews, and various peoples of the Caucasus in the Soviet Union. . . . (p. 1–2).

Macnamara (1967) goes on to point out that Latin America, Africa, and Asia are much more linguistically diverse than Europe. Perhaps the most striking example is India where there are around sixteen major languages, not to mention those of minorities.

Because of our relative isolation geographically and because we are often not aware of the normal multilingual situations in the rest of the world, U.S. knowledge of and attitudes towards bilingualism are quite ethnocentric. Not only are we often unaware of the language complexities in the rest of the world, but our unshaken belief in the American melting pot myth often prevents us from recognizing our own linguistic diversity. The 1970 Bureau of Census of Population Final Report PC(2)-1A, National Origin and Language (p. 492) shows over 7,800,000 native users of Spanish in the U.S.; over 6,000,000 native users of German; over 4,100,000 native users of Italian and over 2,400,000 native users of Polish in the U.S. Polish, incidently, ranks as the fifth foreign language in the U.S. in number of native speakers. In addition, the same report lists an additional twenty-one languages with over 100,000 native users. Anderson and Boyer (1970, Vol. 2, p. 149) also list 43 native American languages that have over 1,000 native users.

The figure for the use of American Sign Language is very difficult to obtain. The chief reason for this is that most surveys of Deaf people do not distinguish between ASL and other types of signing. O'Rourke (1975) estimates that "just under 500,000 deaf persons use sign language." (p. 27). However, this does not give us information on the number of signers who actually use a variety of signing approaching ASL. If we knew, for example, how many of these 500,000 prevocationally Deaf people had Deaf parents, or learned signs before the age of six, or preferred to primarily identify with the Deaf community, etc., we would have a better idea of how many Deaf people use ASL natively. Unfortunately, we do not know all these percentages from the national census of the deaf. Definitely, the number of native ASL users is considerably below 500,000. Our safest bet is to consider that approximately 50% of prevocationally deaf individuals have attended residential school. (Schein and Delk, 1974) The current figure is around 38% (Karchmer and Trybus, 1977) As Meadow (1972) points out, residential schools are the primary place for the enculturation of the majority of Deaf people into the Deaf community. Learning ASL is one way of entering the Deaf community. Thus, we could more safely estimate our *native* users of ASL at around 250,000. O'Rourke (1975) goes on to state "sign language ranks third as a foreign language in the United States." (p. 27). There are several problems with this statement. Sign language is a generic term for several different varieties of two separate languages: ASL and English. One cannot use the term sign language to mean *a* foreign language. Our modest 250,000 estimate should be used for ASL, a language other than English. Second, whether we use the 250,000 people for ASL or O'Rourke's 500,000 figure for sign language, we need to talk about *native* users as the U.S. census does. Neither figure really counts native users. Third, there are nine languages with more than 250,000 *native* users. ASL rates considerably lower than third as a frequently used foreign language in the U.S. We need much better census data, however, before we can say how much lower.

It seems, then, there are definite attitudinal problems facing the implementation of bilingual education for Deaf students. Negative attitudes towards ASL and resultantly towards its use in bilingual education are widespread and long-standing. They are rooted in the American tradition of the melting pot myth and reinforced by the Hearing ethnocentric view that Deaf adults are isolated pathological individuals instead of culturally different members of a suppressed minority group. Participant observers have noted negative attitudes in the Deaf education establishment as well as the Hearing majority culture at large. Such attitudes are especially evident in the decision last year to rule against sign language as a language to be supported under the federal bilingual education funds and in the extremely low desirability and likelihood ratings of acceptance of bilingualism by 122 nationwide experts in deaf education as reported by Prickett and Hunt (1977). Also it is important to remember that these 122 people will be in a position of power and decision-making in deaf education for the next ten years. Acceptance of bilingualism was rated so low that it did not even occur on the scale of likelihood for these people. We have seen, however, from the studies of Diebold (1966) and Paulston (1974) that positive attitudes are more important in success of bilingualism and bilingual education than linguistic concerns are. Obviously, no bilingual program for Deaf individuals will succeed unless (1) all teachers, parents, administrators, children, and local Deaf community members believe that core members of the Deaf community (not just any hearing impaired individuals) should share *equally* in the control, administration, and teaching in any bilingual program or tract for Deaf individuals, and (2) all teachers, parents, administrators, children, and local Deaf community members accept the fact that bilingual education is not compensatory education for Deaf children, i.e., that bilingual education is much more than merely using ASL to get children to where they are ready to use English. ASL must have a respected and important place in education of the Deaf, before a bilingual education program can succeed for Deaf individuals. As we have seen from Prickett and Hunt (1977) neither of these is likely to occur. We should point out here that the hiring of more Deaf teachers in elementary programs on a scale from 1 (most desirable) to 48 (least desirable) ranked 45 out of 48, even lower than acceptance of bilingualism in Prickett and Hunt's (1977) study. Greater hiring of Deaf teachers in elementary schools, which itself is a *prerequisite* for bilingual education, ranks lower in desirability and likelihood in the next ten years than actual acceptance of bilingualism.

Let's suppose for the sake of argument that these negative attitudes will change overnight or at least before the 10 years that Prickett and Hunt forecast for their study. Will it be reasonably easy to establish bilingual education programs, once attitudes change (assuming they can and will)? We are forced to answer, "No, because of the ethnography of communication in the Deaf community."

Problems Due to Ethnography of Communication

As we stated earlier, the ethnography of communication deals with such things as the sociolinguistic influences of participants, topic, setting, channel, and message form and their interrelationships on language preference and use.

The language situation in the Deaf community has been described as diglossic (Stokoe 1970, Woodward 1973a). What concerns us here are primarily setting and participants. As in traditional diglossic situations (see Ferguson 1959), sign language diglossia specifies that the language of education and the classroom be the formal literary variety, in the case of the Deaf community, English. Thus, education normally occurs in the formal variety, especially in lectures. This is true even though the participants are not as comfortable in the formal variety (English) as they are in their conversational variety (ASL). As Ferguson (1964) points out for diglossia in four countries: "To those Americans who would like to evaluate speech in terms of effectiveness of communication, it comes as a shock to discover that many speakers of a language involved in diglossia characteristically prefer to hear a political speech or an expository lecture or a recitation of poetry in H even though it may be less intelligible to them than it would be in L (the conversational variety)." (p. 431–2). The situation in formal education in other countries is very complicated. As Ferguson (1964) indicates: "Although the teachers' use of L (the informal variety) in secondary schools is forbidden by law in some Arab countries, often a considerable part of the teachers' time is taken up with explaining in L (the conversational variety) the meaning of material in H (the formal variety) which has been presented in books or lectures." (p. 431). Those of you familiar with deaf education will recognize the same pattern. If the teacher is Deaf, there will be lecture in English until there is misunderstanding, then the teacher will switch to ASL for explanation. If the teacher is Hearing, you may see students turning to the students who know English and ASL best in a classroom for a "translation" of the Hearing teacher's English into the kind of language the students feel most comfortable with. But even though the Deaf student and Deaf teacher may feel more comfortable with ASL than English, most Deaf students and Deaf teachers will be unable to maintain a total class lecture in ASL. There is too much pressure to switch to English. Gil Eastman (personal communication) reported that he has had pressure from his students to switch to English during his *lectures,* even though they probably understand ASL better. This strong pressure to maintain English in classroom formal presentations is a natural separation of function of languages in the Deaf community. However, it raises some serious problems for the establishment of a bilingual education program. If teachers can't use ASL comfortably and continuously in a classroom, how can both languages achieve equal status and respect in education?

There really is no answer to this question. I suspect that English is preferred because the educational setting is primarily a Hearing social institution. Formal education for the Deaf is controlled by Hearing people. For example, in 1974 only 12% of the educational staff in schools for the Deaf are hearing impaired (and even a smaller percentage of actual Deaf people are classroom teachers). (Kannapell 1974). We have no idea about how many of these hearing impaired individuals are actually sociologically Deaf, that is, they identify with the Deaf community and use ASL.

We cannot really expect that Deaf people will be able to systematically use their own community language, their language of personal identity and group solidarity, in a social institution that is controlled by the Hearing community. (As we will see later, ASL is not shared with Hearing people because it is the language of group solidarity. Languages of group solidarity are not normally used with outsiders, since if they are, they cease to be able to function as a way of identifying people as insiders.)

When Deaf people are accepted as equal in schools for the Deaf and have an equal say in administration as well as classroom teaching, that is, when schools for the Deaf can be viewed by Deaf people as at least equally Deaf and Hearing social institutions or when schools for the Deaf can be viewed by Deaf people as primarily Deaf social institutions, then Deaf people may find it easier to use ASL in classroom to Deaf students, but not before.

However, the change I described above is very unlikely to occur. As we pointed out earlier, Prickett and Hunt (1977) demonstrated that educators in power in the next ten years do not view the hiring of more Deaf elementary teachers as desirable (45 out of 48 rating) or as likely (did not appear on the likelihood table). I don't think that most Deaf people will be willing to start using ASL in the classroom on the premise that this will change attitudes. Why should Deaf people expect that Hearing people will really respect them and their language, when Hearing people discriminate so severely against them in jobs and pay, even within the schools that are supposed to be for them. (Moores 1972).

For example, Schein and Delk (1974) state: "A number of studies have found employers (Hearing) reluctant to hire deaf workers (Rickard, Triandis, and Patterson 1963; Williams 1972). Rickard et al. found general prejudice against hiring disabled applicants. Deafness was rated worse than tuberculosis and wheelchair-bound and better than epilepsy, ex-prison and ex-mental hospital by personnel directors. Similar ratings were given by school administrators, except when the hypothetical applicant sought a position as third-grade teacher. Then the deaf applicant rated worse than all but the epileptic." (p. 89).

While the majority of Deaf people probably cannot quote the Rickard et al. study to support the idea that they have been discriminated against, they have many personal experiences that add up to such discrimination. The negative attitudes of Hearing people and discrimination of Hearing people against Deaf people is probably one of the reasons for the existence of diglossia in the Deaf community. With a seemingly hostile world facing most minority groups in the U.S., there is a feeling among members of the minority group that outsiders must be identified and considered as suspect until they have proved that they do not fit the minority group's stereotype of the majority. There is also a need to identify other members of the minority group so that a feeling of group solidarity can be achieved. Diglossia in principle ensures that most Hearing people will be recognized and stereotyped as Hearing by their signs. (Naturally, there will always be a few exceptions to this trend.) Since the majority of Hearing people do not sign like ASL, they are easily excluded from intimate interaction with Deaf people, who prefer ASL, if Deaf people switch towards English-like signing. This is in fact what happens when Deaf people find out a person is Hearing. (Markowicz and Woodward 1975).

Thus, participants play an important role in language choice in the Deaf community. As long as the diglossic situation exists in the Deaf community, the majority of Hearing people will be prevented from learning ASL, precisely because of the diglossic situation that specifies that English (usually a variety of Pidgin Sign English) be used with Hearing people.

Many Hearing people, including some Hearing linguists, misunderstand the nature and importance of diglossia in the Deaf community. I have had Hearing linguists just beginning to learn to sign tell me, "Oh, I now have a class in ASL. It's fascinating." A few months later, they realize that what they are learning is PSE or even Manual English. Then they start complaining that no Deaf person will teach them ASL no matter how much they beg. The Deaf people keep switching to English. I then suggest that they start taking the time to begin interacting with Deaf people in informal casual situations. Then I suggest that they try to think Deaf and try to imitate the signing of Deaf people to other Deaf people. The Hearing people reply they don't have time and still ask, "Why can't someone teach an ASL class?" If these people really understood Deaf people and the diglossic situation in the Deaf community, they would understand that Deaf ASL is now not appropriate for most classroom situations, especially when the class is full of Hearing people. (I should mention as a note that I was a participant-observer linguist in an experimental class in ASL for Hearing teachers at Gallaudet College. The teacher who was a native signer, who was also undergoing training in linguistics, had to have almost everything prepared before class, so that s/he would not shift into English. Even with all the preparation, there were still shifts that I caught (and undoubtedly many that I missed, since I am not competent to judge what is appropriate in all situations for ASL).

The point of the whole discussion on diglossia, is that diglossia acts as a buffer between Hearing and Deaf communities (Markowicz and Woodward 1975). It allows Hearing people to be identified as outsiders and to be treated carefully before allowing any interaction that could negatively affect the Deaf community. We must remember that Hearing outsiders are stereotyped negatively until they prove themselves to the community. Any Hearing linguist who does not have the time to associate with Deaf people will be viewed as only another "hearie". At the same time, diglossia allows preservation of the language of group identification and solidarity, ASL. Thus diglossia serves as a very positive force in the Deaf community. Successful bilingual education programs must be built around diglossia, that is, they must accommodate diglossia in the community. The best of intentions in cultural change can sometimes be the most devastating. The

Yir Yoront (Sharp 1952) of Australia ceased to exist as a cultural and linguistic group after the introduction of steel axes into the community by missionaries. What the missionaries did not realize was that axes were more than tools; they were symbols of social authority and governed religious organization and ritual. The indiscriminate introduction of steel axes brought about a change so drastic that the society could not handle it. Steel axes in culturally inappropriate hands destroyed the whole social organization of the community.

Diglossia serves important functions in the Deaf community by maintaining social identity and group solidarity. (Markowicz and Woodward 1975). No overt attempts by Hearing people should be made to change the social situation in the Deaf community. Hearing people, almost without exception are outsiders to the Deaf community, and do not necessarily share the values of the Deaf community (De Santis 1976). Plans that Hearing people make for Deaf people can be totally inappropriate because of cultural differences. Thus, if bilingual education is promoted solely by Hearing people, it will probably fail. No social changes, and bilingual education is a social change, should be attempted without adequate knowledge of the possible social ramifications. Sociolinguistic studies of local Deaf·communities are mandatory. These sociolinguistic studies must include (1) studies of attitudes towards the local and/or standard language varieties used and towards bilingual education. (The attitudes of Deaf parents, Deaf students, adult Deaf community members as well as those of Hearing parents and Hearing teachers must be surveyed), (2) an identification of the local sign and oral language varieties used, and (3) a needs assessment of what the school will need to modify in policy, training, and hiring procedures in order to implement a bilingual education program. No school should attempt a bilingual education program or tract without these surveys. Such a sociolinguistic survey is the *first step* in attempting to decide about the feasibility of bilingual education in a given environment. (Saville and Troike 1970). Indiscriminate introduction of bilingual education without the necessary prerequisite sociolinguistic information (described above) could have a detrimental effect on the Deaf community, just as the seemingly beneficial "help" of modern steel tools had a disastrous effect on the Yir Yoront.

So, what can schools do with the diglossic situation? First, schools should try to accommodate the diglossic situation in the classroom. The school should rely on Deaf teachers (core members of the Deaf community, not hearing impaired individuals) to use and teach ASL to Deaf children. This is already normal in the community and it also provides the important argument for hiring more qualified sociologically Deaf teachers to act as role models. Paulston (1974) points out that one of the most positive effects of bilingual education is the providing of positive role models for children from their adult community. Further separation of languages, if desired, could also be made on the basis of subject area. Recent research shows that social studies and history are generally handled in languages other than English in bilingual programs (Saville and Troike 1970). (This is especially true if programs in Deaf awareness, Deaf history, and sign linguistics are developed.) Mathematics and physical science are generally better handled in English (Saville and Troike 1970). This is not because languages other than English cannot handle mathematics or physical science. The reason is that many later mathematics problems that the child will face in college will be "word problems" written in English. Most textbooks in physical science the world over are written in English. While the use of ASL for formal classroom lectures tends to violate the present diglossic situation in the Deaf community, the fact that Deaf teachers will be using ASL to talk about Deaf subjects and current world problems that may face the Deaf student probably will help the Deaf teacher continue signing towards ASL with the students instead of immediately switching to English. There may still be switching problems, however, and if the majority of teachers still tend to switch, it is a sign that the switch is natural and should not be forcibly changed. Other experimental situations can be tried, but *none* should be forced.

As should be obvious, obtaining through training and/or recruitment *qualified* teachers and teacher aides is not easy but extremely necessary for the success of such a program. Saville and Troike (1970) strongly emphasize that: "a teacher is not adequately qualified to teach a language merely because it is his native tongue. The following requirements should be considered by those hiring teachers for bilingual education programs:

- willingness to participate in an innovative program.
- knowledge of the structures of both languages of instruction.
- general understanding of the nature of language, including the acceptability and inevitability of dialect variations in all living languages.
- specific understanding of his own dialect and dialect of the area in which he teaches.
- knowledge of methods for teaching a second language.
- understanding and acceptance of all cultures represented in the community.
- knowledge of the growth and development patterns of children.
- competence to provide a good linguistic model, preferably in both languages. If a teacher is competent in only one language, he should be placed in a team teaching situation, and should not teach in his weak language." (p. 26).

Problems of Bilingualism in the Deaf Community

A number of people have commented that there is bilingualism in the Deaf community in the U.S. (Stokoe 1970, 1972, Kannapell 1974, 1977, Woodward and Markowicz 1975). It is extremely important to distinguish two types of bilingualism: individual and societal bilingualism. Individual bilingualism refers to the individual's competence in more than one language; societal bilingualism refers to the fact that while two or more languages may be used in a community, many individuals may not be competent in the two languages. While a number of researchers have emphasized the individual bilingualism of Deaf children of Deaf parents, we should be aware that bilingualism is basically a societal phenomenon in the Deaf community, not an individual one. The majority of Deaf individuals are not competent in English, although all individuals can move somewhat along the continuum between ASL and English.

As the National Center for Law and the Deaf's 1977 request for bilingual education pointed out:

> The difficulties that deaf students have in learning English have been particularly well documented. No studies have shown deaf people to have the same competence in English as hearing people. Furth (1966) reported that only 12% of deaf students between the ages of 15.5 and 16.5 have reading levels at fourth grade or higher. Several studies of over 400 deaf students found that 10 year old hearing students had better English syntactic competence than 18 year old deaf students in relative clauses (Quigley and Wilbur, 1974), verbal complements (Quigley, Wilbur, and Montanelli, in press) conjoining (Wilbur, Montanelli, and Quigley, 1976).
>
> Other studies investigating deaf students' English competence from the framework of a deviant form of English (Myklebust, 1964; Perry, 1968), of transformational grammar (Schmitt, 1968; Power and Quigley, 1973; Quigley, Smith and Wilbur, 1974), and of English as a second language for deaf students (Charrow and Fletcher, 1974) have all shown that the majority of deaf students do not have native competence in English. (p. 1–2).

We are thus faced with a bilingual education situation where the majority of students entering schools for the deaf have no competence in either of the two languages of instruction. They may in fact have developed their own language, separate from ASL and English (Feldman and Goldin-Meadow 1975). The entering students who do have competence in ASL are very small, probably about 4–6% of the total population (Deaf of two Deaf parents). If we assume that Deaf children of Deaf parents who have some college education will probably be the most likely candidates for being bilingual in ASL and English, we are probably talking about a smaller percentage of the Deaf population for school age children, since not all Deaf children of two Deaf parents attend college. (Woodward 1977, 1978).

Thus a bilingual education program will have to have separate educational materials for students who are already competent in ASL as compared with those who are not and separate educational materials for students who are already competent in English as compared with those who are not. This is at least four sets of materials. This will require a great deal of curriculum development. In fact, it also necessitates a good deal of sociolinguistic research before adequate materials can be developed. It would be important to know, for example, what kinds of language competence students enter with when they are not competent in ASL or English. Otherwise, we are faced with the problem of teaching basic skills in ASL to some students, while other students are ready for the kind of instruction we give natively competent students in poetry, history of the language, folklore, public lecturing, etc. We face the same kind of problems in English also. If we do not have separate materials, we are faced with boring and suppressing the interest of the minority of fluent users because of materials that are too easy or faced with overwhelming the majority of students who are not fluent because of materials that are far too complicated for their linguistic competence in the language(s) in question.

Actually, we are faced with this problem of separate materials development in monolingual education programs in English. The point is that everyone has tended to ignore the problem. Undoubtedly, part of the present educational problems in schools for the deaf is the wide difference of students' language background. The additional problems in a bilingual education program are that materials need to be developed in two languages. This may be too much for some schools. As we mentioned before in the introduction, if bilingual education programs are set up and do not succeed, we may be faced with the prospect of returning to strict oralism, a sociolinguistic situation considerably worse than what exists now. Given the attitudinal and additional sociolinguistic complications in the sign language situation in the U.S., only those schools that have the adequate resources in linguists, administrators, teachers, parents, children, and adult Deaf community members should attempt to set up bilingual programs or tracts. There are other improvements that can be made in schools without adequate resources. (We will discuss some of these in the conclusion.)

Problems of the Sign Language Continuum

Up to this point, we have discussed problems related to negative attitudes towards ASL and bilingual education, problems of diglossia, and problems of the types of bilingualism already existing in the Deaf community. We are now faced with a new problem. What is ASL? The language situation in the Deaf community has been described as a bilingual-diglossic *continuum* between ASL and English, with pidgin-like varieties in between. These pidgin-like varieties have received various names by some people: Ameslish (Bragg 1973), Siglish (Fant 1972), Signed English (O'Rourke 1970), Manual English (Stokoe 1970) and Pidgin Sign English (or PSE) (Woodward 1972, 1973d). The proliferation of names is unfortunate. First it confuses teachers and it obscures the idea of a continuum. I have heard that some people are saying that PSE is a separate language from ASL and English. While it is true that PSE is different from pure ASL and from pure English, it is not a separate language. There is no empirical way in the world to define where PSE begins and ends. PSE was used specifically to handle the situation that exists between ASL and English. Namely that there is no clearcut empirically definable division between ASL and English. PSE merely describes the fact there is no clearcut division and allows one to talk about English-y ASL and ASL-like English for Deaf people and ASL-like English for a few Hearing people and English-y English for most Hearing people.

Although there is no clearcut division between ASL and English, there are empirical ways to describe the continuum. Woodward (1973a, b, c, 1974, 1976) handles the description of variation through sociolinguistic variation theory (implicational scales and variable rules). Through these techniques, it is possible to demonstrate statistically that Deaf signers tend to use more ASL-like signing than Hearing people (Woodward 1973b), that Deaf people with Deaf parents use more ASL-like signing than Deaf people with Hearing parents (Woodward 1973a), that people who learned signs before the age of six will use more ASL-like signing than people who learned signs after the age of six (Woodward 1973b), and that college is an important variable (Woodward 1973b). Anderson (current research) has pointed out that the original conclusion of the independent variable of college education was misleading. If signers are subdivided into those having Deaf parents and those having Hearing parents and then the variable of college is introduced, Deaf people of Deaf parents who attend college use less ASL than Deaf people of Hearing parents who attend college. Gallaudet then can be seen as reducing ASL use for Deaf of Deaf parents and increasing it for Deaf of Hearing parents. Not all ASL rules were equally affected by these social variables. For example, frequency of Agent-Beneficiary directionality use was related to deafness, age of sign language acquisition and education (Woodward 1973a), while verb reduplication was related to these three factors *and* the factor of parentage. (Woodward 1973b).

This brings us to a crucial point. Most of the linguistic studies of ASL have not described their informants (usually only one or two) and have not described any empirical ways that they attempted to verify that what they were getting was close to "pure" ASL signing. Such contradictory claims as previous SOV and present predominant SVO word order in ASL (Fischer 1975), free word order in ASL (Friedman 1975), or preferred SVO with variant word orders depending on facial adverbials (Liddell 1978) could be more easily resolved with a large scale study utilizing variation theory. It should be pointed out that there are few consultants in each of these studies, that linguistic consultants in each of these studies are non-Southeastern, White, Middle class (in the Deaf community), and in at least two of the studies, college-educated. (This same trend for selection of consultants can be found in almost all studies of ASL.) If one performed the same studies on a large sample, especially in the South and more especially among Black signers, it is very likely that one would find a greater use of the historically older verb final order among Southeastern consultants and within Southeastern consultants, Blacks might very well use more of the historically older verb final orders than Whites of the same age. This is a reasonable hypothesis, since with the exception of assimilation of compound handshapes, (see Woodward and Erting 1975), Southeasterners tend to retain older forms more often than Northerners (Woodward 1976, Woodward and De Santis 1977b). Also in the South, Blacks use historically older forms more often than Whites of the same age (Woodward and Erting 1975, Woodward 1976, Woodward and De Santis 1977b).

The moral of the story is that we may very well know much less about the structure of ASL as it is used by the majority of Deaf consultants than we think we do. As I mentioned earlier, most studies only look at Deaf children of Deaf parents, about 4%–6% of the Deaf population. In addition, they have tended to focus on White Deaf people who are not from the Southeast U.S. This brings our population figures down somewhat (3–4.5%). What brings them down again is that many of the Deaf people of two Deaf parents who have been studied have been college-educated. Remembering Anderson's point that Deaf people of two Deaf parents who attend some college tend to be less like pure ASL than those who did not, we have the very serious situation of not only ignoring the majority of the Deaf community in most linguistic research, but of describing a type of ASL whose use is extremely restricted.

The solution to this problem is to test out these studies that have the above problems on a fairly large sample of consultants from varying regional, social, ethnic, and age backgrounds. As we have pointed out research in all of these variables significantly and independently influence ASL use. To give a brief illustration here of how complex the situation can be: regional, social, ethnic, and age and historical variations are often related. For example, Woodward and De Santis (1977b) have shown that French signers utilized more of the older two-handed signs on the face than American signers ($x^2 = 52.01$, df $= 1$, p<.001). In the same study, it was pointed out that Southerners used the older two-handed signs more often than Northerners. In the South, older Whites used the older two-handed signs more often than younger Whites ($x^2 = 5.17$, df $= 1$, p$<$.05). Also in the South, younger Blacks paralleled older Whites, that is, they used older two-handed signs on the face more often than younger Whites ($x^2 = 6.89$, df $= 1$, p$<$.01).

On the whole, such variation has been misunderstood in deaf education with the result that problems have arisen in language attitudes and tolerance. These problems in attitudes and tolerance will also be problems in bilingual education.

Problems of Regional, Social, Ethnic, and Historical Variation in Signing

Variation, since it is normal and to be expected, should pose no problems for any kind of language education, monolingual or multilingual. However, it invariably does cause problems. The problems arise because of the mistaken idea that language, in general, and English, in particular, does not vary but is like a whole entity that quite obviously everyone must use the same way. Part of this arises from our orthography., For example, we see the word "d-o-g". If we are literate, we understand the word, and also pronounce it. However, there are numerous variations in the pronunciation that we may not be aware of: dag, dɔg, dawg, duǝg, etc.

No problem in communication occurs, if our way of using a language is not too different from the way of the person that we are communicating with. Problems arise when the differences are great, and/or when we haven't been exposed to the differences for a sufficient time to become adjusted to them. However, problems in language education can occur even when communication of content is easy. Teachers in most language classrooms are not at all tolerant of language differences of their students. The immediate temptation is to eradicate those differences, instead of appreciating them and using them to teach the students about the intricacies of language behavior.

Sign languages are discriminated against because they are a different code *and* channel from the majority oral language. Thus Deaf people have an extremely difficult time finding anyone who actually respects their language (and not just says they do). Moreover, many Hearing people who are not native to any type of signing will put down any diffferences they see in signing. Many Deaf ASL users have only slightly more positive attitudes towards differences in signing. I have had Deaf people deny that specific examples of signs I have given are actually used by any Deaf people. When I tell them when and where I recorded the signs or even show them the signs on videotape, they say "Well, they are lazy." or "That's still not the proper sign." or "They are just using home signs."

With attitudes like these, it is no wonder that teachers tend to repress local varieties, especially those of ethnic minorities like Blacks.

"I once asked a (Deaf) Black woman receiving vocational training when she learned signs. She replied that her interpreter just taught her. Being surprised by her fluency, I asked if she hadn't attended a residential school. She said yes. I then continued with, 'You mean you didn't use signs at the residential school?' She answered, 'Yes, but now I'm learning correct signs.' " (Woodward 1976, p. 217).

Now just who told her that she wasn't using "proper" signs? Certainly not her peer group. It is obvious that her interpreter and/or former teachers told her. This situation is not rare, but widespread.

If bilingual/bicultural education for Deaf individuals is to succeed, the teacher must know and use the students' language variety. Otherwise, the student may very well be faced (like some Hearing Chicano children in the Southwest) with having to learn not only one foreign language (English) but the other language in the so-called bilingual school—textbook Spanish for the Hearing Chicano or "Gallaudet" signing for the Deaf child. More importantly, ignoring regional, social and ethnic variations in signing may make the student aware that the school does not respect or at least does not care about his/her social identity. A Deaf or Hearing person who ignores the local community's signs is making a similar mistake to a Hearing person who ignores ASL.

In fact, knowledge, use, and respect of all signing varieties could be of use in selecting vocabulary for ASL use. For example, many people in Washington, D.C. do not have signs for "truck", "shoelace", "turnip greens" . . . and yet teachers and students may want a sign. Instead of inventing an artificial sign on the spur of the moment, it seems much more reasonable to borrow a sign from another community. Black Southern signers have signs for "truck", "shoelace", "turnip greens", etc.

Kendall School in its ASL and English language policy has recognized the need to recognize and respect students' language varieties. Where the school children and the local Deaf community do not have a sign (in ASL or English) for a specific idea, signs from other regions of the country (including all ethnic groups) are borrowed.

What I am trying to say is that good policies for language use in school, that is, those policies that demand tolerance and acceptance of language variation, must come from sociolinguistic research. While I don't agree completely with Kendall's policy (especially as it relates to English), it is the most enlightened language policy I have seen for deaf education. It will not be difficult for individual schools to imitate such a policy for ASL and English. However, no one school can borrow Kendall's ASL or English signs wholesale because there probably are other types of signs being locally used. Thus, it would be contradictory to borrow Kendall's policy *and* signs, since the policy specifies the ASL and English signs are based on the language of the children in the D.C. area. If these signs are not used in another community, it violates the rights of that particular Deaf community to use them under an official language policy.

Sociolinguistic descriptions of the local Deaf community are needed; however, this requires time, money, effort, and cooperation of the individual school. As I stated in the introduction, from the actions of the Office of Education, and from Prickett and Hunt's (1977) study, most schools are not willing to make such a commitment to accept and study the local varieties of signing. If this is true, then successful bilingual education for Deaf children is a long way off. How can anyone expect a bilingual program to succeed where a monolingual one fails, if *both* language varieties have to be learned by the children instead of just one? Without respect for and positive attitudes towards the child's language variety, we can also expect less language learning on the part of the student and a generally poorer performance in education (Paulston 1974).

Conclusion

Bilingual education is a very desirable alternative in the education of Deaf students, however, there are a number of very large and important problems for most schools in setting up bilingual education programs for Deaf students. Core members of the Deaf community (not just hearing impaired individuals) must share equally in the control, administration, and teaching in any bilingual program or tract for Deaf individuals. The bilingual program must allow the free use of American Sign Language in and for itself and not merely as a temporary tool for teaching English. Negative attitudes on the part of teachers, parents, administrators, students, and the local Deaf community must be overcome. The recent decision by the Office of Education and the projected future of education of the deaf for the next ten years (Prickett and Hunt 1977) would indicate that the problem of negative attitudes is severe. The school must then face the problem of designing the bilingual program or tract to conform to the existing diglossic situation in the Deaf community. Separate materials and teaching techniques will have to be used for students with different competencies in ASL and English. Our information on ASL is limited by the fact that most studies have not considered variation and have studied consultants who are not representative of the majority of members in the Deaf community. Furthermore, there have been traditional ignorance of and negative attitudes towards regional, social, ethnic and historical variations in ASL and English. Further research in these areas is needed as well as a change in attitudes.

Relating to all problem areas discussed in this paper, Deaf teachers should be chosen wherever possible from *core members of the local Deaf community* since they will probably best know specific sign varieties used in their area. The people must also be willing to use these varieties. In addition, if there are ethnic minority students, an effort should be made locally to find Deaf teachers from the same backgrounds. More than likely, all these prospective Deaf teachers will also have to be enrolled by the school in teacher training programs simultaneously, since they undoubtedly will not have the proper credentials. Such training, however, may be much easier than the alternative of finding (or training) Hearing teachers (to be) competent in ASL. As Vorih and Rosier (1978) point out in their discussion of the *successful* Rock Point Navaho-English bilingual program: "It was felt it would be far easier to prepare Navaho aides to teach than it would be to teach certified Anglo teachers to speak Navaho, *so Navaho aides were trained on site.*" (p. 268).

Hearing people should be taught the local variety of signs appropriate for Hearing people in that locale. They should also be able to recognize local ethnic and sex variations in signs. Attitude training towards the areas discussed in this paper and other areas as well as training in sign linguistics (and preferably Deaf culture) will be necessary for all Hearing teachers and perhaps for a large number of Deaf teachers, also.

Obviously, all of this necessitates massive changes in the school's social system, which are unlikely to come very quickly. Thus it is probably not reasonable to expect that a whole school could adopt a totally bilingual program in a reasonable amount of time. Given relative independence from and acceptance by other tracts in the school, (and that is a large variable), it would be more reasonable to expect that the school could adopt a bilingual tract. However, the problems in a bilingual tract will be the same as in a bilingual program but not as massive. There are still additional problems like students moving in and/or out of the tract.

Saville and Troike (1970) suggest that "the following qualifications should be considered in the hiring of a program coordinator:

- Is he a fluent speaker of both languages?
- Is he sensitive to public relations?
- Does he understand children, schools, linguistics, anthropology, psychology, curriculum design, evaluation, and the principles of research?

The position of coordinator is as demanding as the qualifications suggest, since he will be *responsible for:*

- recommending principles, objectives, and program organization to the school board.
- recruiting bilingual teachers, aides, consultants, and other personnel.
- conducting pre-service and in-service training of teachers and aides.
- curriculum design.
- materials preparation, selection, and adaptation.
- plan of evaluation.

- contacts with state and federal agencies concerned.
- public relations." (p. 21).

It is quite doubtful that such a person exists for any school to hire. However, rather than settling for the best unqualified individual, a *small* panel of experts in crucial fields can be established to carry out the above-mentioned actions.

Certainly, bilingual education, while desirable, is not going to be an easy or cheap proposition. In fact, most schools will probably not be able or willing to make the necessary commitments to research, teacher training, etc. that a shift to bilingual education would mean. This, however, does not mean that the schools can do nothing. The schools themselves can pave the way for the real possibility of bilingual education, by adopting some changes within their current set-up. Schools can establish attitude awareness training to help begin changing some of the stereotypes of Deaf people and ASL. The school can encourage the acceptance of ASL outside and inside the classroom in appropriate sociolinguistic situations. Schools can make a commitment to hire many more qualified core members of the Deaf community to work as teachers, administrators, and helpers in the school system. Schools can also invite adult members of the Deaf community to come into the schools to explain to the students (and parents) what kinds of problems and pleasures Deaf people face OUT-WORLD. Schools can encourage research especially on the local varieties of signing (including ethnic minorities) by qualified researchers. By qualified, I mean Deaf and Hearing persons trained strongly in linguistics. I do not mean hiring someone who has had a couple of courses in linguistics.

By doing the above and much more, the schools can actually cause a situation to evolve where bilingual education could naturally happen. Again I want to stress the uselessness and danger of setting up poorly designed bilingual programs. They can only fail because of poor attitudes and administration. In addition, and more importantly, they will damage the image of successful programs and skew the results of research evaluations of bilingual education. Bilingual education, like total communication properly defined, is not a panacea. Please don't jump on any bandwagons before you are ready. One can get hurt and hurt others in the process.

References

Anderson, T. and M. Boyer. 1970. *Bilingual Schooling in the United States.* Austin, TX: Southwest Educational Development Laboratory.

Bailey, C. 1973. *Variation and Linguistic Theory.* Washington, D.C.: Center for Applied Linguistics.

Baker, C. 1975. Regulators and Turn-taking in American Sign Language. Paper presented at the 50th Annual Meeting of the Linguistic Society of America.

Battison, R. 1974. Phonological Deletion in American Sign Language. *Sign Language Studies*, 5, 1–19.

Battison, R. and I.K. Jordan. 1976. Cross Cultural Communication With Foreign Signers: Fact and Fancy. *Sign Language Studies*, 10, 53–68.

Battison, R., H. Markowicz, and J. Woodward. 1975. A Good Rule of Thumb: Variable Phonology in American Sign Language. In Shuy, R. and R. Fasold, eds. *Analyzing Variation in Language*. Washington, D.C.: Georgetown University Press.

Bellugi, U. and E. Klima. 1975. Aspects of Sign Language and Its Structure. In Kavanagh and Cutting, eds. *The Role of Speech in Language*. Cambridge: MIT Press, 171–205.

Bickerton, D. 1973. The Structure of Polylectal Grammars. *Georgetown University MSLL*, 25, 17–42.

Bornstein, H. 1973. A Description of Some Current Sign Systems Designed to Represent English. *American Annals of the Deaf*, 118, 454-463.

Bragg, B. 1973. Ameslish: Our National Heritage. *American Annals of the Deaf*, 118, 672–674.

Charrow, V. 1974. Deaf English: An Investigation of the Written English Competence of Deaf Adolscents. Unpublished Ph.D. dissertation, Stanford University.

Charrow, V. and J. Fletcher. 1974. English as the Second Language of Deaf Children. *Developmental Psychology*, 10:4, 463–470.

Croneberg, C. 1965. The Linguistic Community. In Stokoe, W., D. Casterline. and C. Croneberg. *A Dictionary of American Sign Language*. Washington D.C.: Gallaudet College Press.

De Santis, S. 1976. The Deaf Community in the United States. Working paper, Linguistics Research Lab, Gallaudet College, Washington, D.C.

De Santis, S. 1977. Elbow to Hand Shift in French and American Sign Languages. A paper presented at the annual NWAVE conference, Georgetown University, Washington, D.C., October.

Diebold, A. 1966. The Consequences of Early Bilingualism in Cognitive Development and Personality Formation. ERIC No. ED 020 491.

Erting, C. 1978. Language Policy and Deaf Ethnicity in the United States. *Sign Language Studies*, 19, 139–152.

Fant, L. 1972. *Ameslan*. Silver Spring, MD.: National Association of the Deaf.

Fasold, R. 1970. Two Models of Socially Significant Linguistic Variation. *Language*, 46, 551–563.

Fay, A. 1898. *Marriages of the Deaf in America*. Washington;, D.C.: Volta Bureau.

Feldman, H. and S. Goldin-Meadow. 1975. The Creation of a Communication System: A Study of Deaf Children of Hearing Parents. *Sign Language Studies*, 8, 225–234.

Ferguson, C. 1959. Diglossia. *Word*, 15, 325–340. (Reprinted in Hymes, D. 1964. *Language in Culture and Society*. New York: Harper and Row.)

Fischer, S. 1975. Influences on Word Order Change in American Sign Language. In Li, C. *Word Order and Word Order Change*. Austin, Texas: University of Texas Press.

Fishman, J. 1961. Tsveyshprakhikayt in a Yidisher Shul: Einike Korelatn un Nitkorelatn. *Bleter far Yidisher Dertsiung*, 4, 32–42.

Fishman, J. 1967. Bilingualism With and Without Diglossia: Diglossia With and Without Bilingualism. *Journal of Social Issues*, 23:2.

Friedman, L. 1975. The Manifestation of Subject and Object in American Sign Language. A paper presented at the Annual Meeting of the Linguistic Society of America, San Francisco, December.

Frishberg, N. 1975. Arbitrariness and Iconicity: Historical Change in American Sign Language. *Language*, 51, 696–719.

Furth, H. 1966. A Comparison of Reading Test Norms of Deaf and Hearing Children. *American Annals of the Deaf*, 111, 461–462.

Gali, A. 1928. Comment Measurer L'influence du Bilinguisme. In Bureau International D'Education: *Le Bilinguisme et L' education*. Geneva. (See Weinreich, 1968.)

Hymes, D. 1964. Towards Ethnographies of Communication. In Gumperz, J. and D. Hymes. eds. *The Ethnography of Communication, American Anthropologist*, 66, 6, part 2, 1–34.

Hymes, D. 1971. Pidginization and Creolization of Languages. Cambridge: Cambridge University Press.

John, V. and V. Horner. 1961. Early Childhood Bilingual Education. New York: MLA-ACTFL.

Johnston, G. 1977. George's Scope: The Confusing Terminology: Crisis for 1977, 1978, 1979, etc. *The Deaf Spectrum*, 20–25.

Kannapell, B. 1974. Bilingual Education: A New Direction in the Education of the Deaf. *The Deaf American*, 26, 10, 9–15.

Kannapell, B. 1977. The Deaf Person as a Teacher of American Sign Language. A paper presented at the First NSSLRT meeting, Chicago.

Karchmer, M. and R. Trybus. 1977. Who Are the Deaf Children in 'Mainstream' Programs? Washington, D.C.: Gallaudet College, Office of Demographic Studies.

Klima, E. and U. Bellugi. 1975. Wit and Poetry in American Sign Language. *Sign Language Studies*, 8, 203–224.

Labov, W. 1969. Contraction, Deletion, and Inherent Variability of the English Copula. *Language*, 45, 715–762.

Labov, W. 1972. *Sociolinguistic Patterns*. Philadelphia: University of Pennsylvania Press.

Lambert, W. 1978. Some Cognitive and Socio-cultural Consequences of Being Bilingual. A paper presented at the Georgetown Round Table on Languages and Linguistics, Washington, D.C.

Liddell, S. 1975. Restrictive Relative Clauses in American Sign Language. A paper presented at the Summer meeting of the Linguistic Society of America. Urbana-Champaign.

Long, K. and A. Padilla. 1970. Evidence for Bilingual Antecedents of Academic Success in a Group of Spanish-American College Students. Unpublished research report, Western Washington State College.

Macnamara, J., ed. 1967. Problems of Bilingualism. *The Journal of Social Issues*, 23:2.

Malherbe, E. 1934. The Bilingual School: A Study of Bilingualism in South Africa, Johannesburg. (See Weinreich, 1968.)

Markowicz, H. 1972. Some Sociolinguistic Considerations of American Sign Language. *Sign Language Studies*, 1, 15–41.

Markowicz, H. and J. Woodward. 1975 (1978, 1982). Language and the Maintenance of Ethnic Boundaries in the Deaf Community. A paper presented at the Conference on Culture and Communication, Temple University, Philadelphia, March. Published in *Communication and Cognition* and in this volume.

Marose, S. 1977. Sign Language Aids Deaf Kids to Speak. *The Deaf Spectrum*, 1–2.

Meadow, K. 1972. Sociolinguistics, Sign Language, and the Deaf Subculture. In O'Rourke, T. *Psycholinguistics and Total Communication: The State of the Art.* Silver Spring, MD.: American Annals of the Deaf.

Moores, D. 1972. Communication: Some Unanswered Questions and Some Unquestioned Answers. In O'Rourke, T. *Psycholinguistics and Total Communication: The State of the Art.* Silver Spring, MD.: American Annals of the Deaf.

Myklebust, H. 1960. *The Psychology of Deafness: Sensory Deprivation, Learning, and Adjustment.* New York: Grune and Stratton.

National Center for Law and the Deaf. 1977. Formal Request to Department of Health, Education, and Welfare, Office of Education, Office of General Counsel for Elementary and Secondary Schools that Sign Language be Considered a Language for Use in Bilingual Study Projects Under the Bilingual Education Act, Title VII of the Elementary and Secondary Education Act of 1965 (20 USC 8806), April 22, 1977.

O'Rourke, T. 1970. Quotation in Stokoe, W. 1970. *The Study of Sign Language.* Arlington, VA.: Center for Applied Linguistics.

O'Rourke, T. 1975. National Association of the Deaf Communicative Skills Program *Programs for the Handicapped.* Washington, D.C.: Dept. of Health, Education, and Welfare, Office for Handicapped Individuals, April 15.

Padden, C. and H. Markowicz. 1975 (1976). Crossing Cultural Group Boundaries Into the Deaf Community. A paper presented at the Conference on Culture and Communication, Temple University, Philadelphia, March. Published in 1976 as Cultural Conflicts Between Hearing and Deaf Communities. In F.B. and A.B. Crammatte. eds. *Proceedings of the VII World Congress of the World Federation of the Deaf.* Washington, D.C.: National Association of the Deaf.

Padilla, A. and K. Long. 1969. As Assessment of Successful Spanish-American Students at the University of New Mexico. Paper presented to the annual meeting of the AAAS Rocky Mountain Division, Colorado Springs.

Paulston, C. 1974. Implications of Language Learning Theory for Language Planning. Arlington, VA.: Center for Applied Linguistics. *Papers in Applied Linguistics, Bilingual Education Series,* 1.

Peal, E. and W. Lambert. 1962. The Relation of Bilingualism to Intelligence. *Psychological Monographs: General and Applied.* LXXVI, 27, 1–23.

Perry, F. 1968. The Psycholinguistic Abilities of Deaf Children: An Exploratory Investigation II. *Australian Teacher of the Deaf,* 9, 153–160.

Power, D. and S. Quigley. 1973. Deaf Children's Acquisition of the Passive Voice. *Journal of Speech and Hearing Research,* 17, 325–341.

Prickett, H. and J. Hunt. 1977. Education of the Deaf—The Next Ten Years. *American Annals of the Deaf,* 122:4, 365–381.

Quigley, S., D. Montanelli, and R. Wilbur. Some Aspects of the Verbal System in the Language of Deaf Students. *Journal of Speech and Hearing Research,* in press.

Quigley, S., N. Smith and R. Wilbur. 1974. Comprehension of Relativized Sentences by Deaf Students. *Journal of Speech and Hearing Research.*

Rainer, J., K. Altschuler, and F. Kallman. 1963. *Family and Mental Health in a Deaf Population*. New York: State Psychiatric Institute, Columbia University.

Rickard, T., E. Triandis, and C. Patterson. 1963. Indices of Employer Prejudice Toward Disabled Applicants. *Journal of Applied Psychology*, 47, 52–55.

Saer, D. 1923. The Effect of Bilingualism on Intelligence. *British Journal of Psychology*, 14, 25–38.

Samarin, W. 1971. Salient and Substantive Pidginization. In Hymes, D. *Pidginization and Creolization of Languages*. Cambridge: Cambridge University Press. 117–140.

Saville, M. and R. Troike. 1970. *A Handbook of Bilingual Education*. Arlington, VA.: Center for Applied Linguistics.

Schein, J. and M. Delk. 1974. *The Deaf Population of the United States*. Silver Spring, MD.: National Association of the Deaf.

Schmitt, P. 1968. Deaf Children's Comprehension and Production of Sentence Transformations and Verb Tenses. Unpublished Ph.D. dissertation, University of Illinois.

Sharp, L. 1952. Steel Axes for Stone-age Aborigines. *Human Organization*, 2, 17–22.

Stokoe, W. 1960. *Sign Language Structure: An Outline of the Visual Communication System of the American Deaf*. University of Buffalo, Occasional Paper 8.

Stokoe, W. 1970. Sign Language Diglossia. *Studies in Linguistics*, 21, 27–41.

Stokoe, W. 1972. *Semiotics and Human Sign Languages*. Mouton: The Hague.

Stokoe, W. 1973. Sign Language Syntax and Human Language Capacity. A forum lecture at the Summer LSA Institute, Ann Arbor.

Stokoe, W. and R. Battison. 1975. Sign Language, Mental Health, and Satisfying Interaction. A paper presented at the First National Symposium on Mental Health Needs of Deaf Adults and Youth. (To appear in the proceedings of the conference.)

U.S. Bureau of the Census. 1973. Census of Population, 1970, Subject Reports, Final Report PC(2)-1A, National Origin and Language.

Vorih, L. and P. Rosier. 1978. Rock Point Community School: An Example of a Navajo-English Bilingual Elementary School Program. *TESOL Quarterly*, 12, 3, 263–9.

Weinreich, U. 1968. *Languages in Contact*. The Hague: Mouton.

Wilbur, R., S. Quigley, and D. Montanelli. 1975. Conjoined Structures in the Written Language of Deaf Students. *Journal of Speech and Hearing Research*, 18, 319–335.

Wilbur, R., D. Montanelli, and S. Quigley. 1976. Pronominalization in the Language of Deaf Students. *Journal of Speech and Hearing Research*, 19, 120–140.

Williams, C. 1972. Is Hiring the Handicapped Good Business? *Journal of Rehabilitation*, March–April, 30–34.

Woodward, J. 1972. Implications for Sociolinguistic Research Among the Deaf. *Sign Language Studies*, 1, 1–7.

Woodward, J. 1973a. Implicational Lects on the Deaf Diglossic Continuum. Unpublished Ph.D. dissertation, Georgetown University.

Woodward, J. 1973b. Some Observations on Sociolinguistic Variation and American Sign Language. *Kansas Journal of Sociology*, 9:2, 191–200.

Woodward, J. 1973c. Interrule Implication in American Sign Language. *Sign Language Studies*, 3, 47–56.

Woodward, J. 1973d. Some Characteristics of Pidgin Sign English. *Sign Language Studies*, 3, 39–46.

Woodward, J. 1974. A Report on Montana-Washington Implicational Research. *Sign Language Studies*, 4, 77–101.

Woodward, J. 1976. Black Southern Signing. *Language in Society*, 5:2, 211–218.

Woodward, J. 1977. English Language Program Survey of Incoming Preps, Gallaudet College.

Woodward, J. 1978. English Language Program Survey of Incoming Preps, Gallaudet College.

Woodward, J. 1979. *Signs of Sexual Behavior*. Silver Spring, MD: T.J. Publishers.

Woodward, J. and S. De Santis. 1977a Negative Incorporation in French and American Sign Languages. *Language in Society*, 6:3, 379–388.

Woodward, J. and S. De Santis. 1977b. Two to One It Happens: Dynamic Phonology in Two Sign Languages. *Sign Language Studies*, 17, 329–346.

Woodward, J. and C. Erting. 1975. Synchronic Variation and Historical Change in American Sign Language. *Language Sciences*, 37, 9–12.

Woodward, J., C. Erting, and S. Oliver. 1976. Facing and Hand(l)ing Variation in American Sign Language. *Sign Language Studies*, 10, 43–52.

Woodward, J. and H. Markowicz. 1975 (1980). Some Handy New Ideas on Pidgins and Creoles: Pidgin Sign Languages. A paper presented at the 1975 International Conference on Pidgin and Creole Languages, Honolulu, January. Published in Stokoe, W. ed. *Sign and Culture*, Silver Spring, MD.: Linstok Press.

Zappert, L. and R. Cruz. 1977. *Bilingual Education: An Appraisal of Empirical Research*. Berkeley, California: Bay Area Bilingual Education League/Lau Center, Berkeley Unified School District.

James Woodward

Beliefs About and Attitudes Toward Deaf People and Sign Language on Providence Island

Introduction

Most societies researched to date view Deaf people as inferior to Hearing people and often actively discriminate against Deaf individuals and groups and their sign languages. However the three thousand Hearing people on Providence Island come closer to an equal acceptance of Deaf people and sign language than do those in most other societies that have been studied.

This study was undertaken to help determine the reliability of field observations made by researchers that there were relatively positive attitudes toward Deaf people and toward sign language on Providence Island, where the incidence of deafness in the population is two to three times the expected number (cf. Washabaugh, Woodward, and De Santis 1978).

We have interviewed Hearing people from most of the major villages on the island to record articulated beliefs about (1) marriage, mental abilities, occupational equality, and social integration of Deaf people and (2) the origins of Providence Island Sign Language, universality and uniqueness of sign language, the grammar of Providence Island Sign Language, the effectiveness of communication in Providence Island Sign Language, and the right of Deaf people to use a sign language. These beliefs give insights into attitudes toward Deaf people and sign language.

After a brief description of the respondents and data collection, responses to questions in the above areas are analyzed and are compared and contrasted with typical attitudes in the educational establishment for the deaf in the U.S.

Respondents and Data

We have surveyed five of the eight major villages on Providence: F.B., L.H., O.T., M., and R.P. No Deaf people live or have lived in F.B., but one

Deaf person from a third village has worked occasionally in F.B. L.H., O.T., and R.P. have a long tradition of Deaf people and Deaf and Hearing signers. M. in contrast has two younger deaf people who do not seem to prefer to sign. One Hearing adult from each house in F.B. was interviewed. In L.H., one adult from every second house was interviewed. The sample for O.T. was one Hearing adult from every fifth house; for M. and R.P. the sample was one Hearing adult from every tenth house.

Table 1 shows the background information of the 57 respondents. Slightly less than half the respondents are males. We had hoped to obtain the

TABLE 1

Background Information on Providence Island Respondents.

Respondent	Village	Sex	Signing Ability (self reported)	Contact with Deaf People
1	F.B.	M	good	a lot
2	F.B.	F	good	a lot
3	F.B.	M	fair	some
4	F.B.	F	very good	all the time
5	F.B.	F	poor	a little
6	F.B.	F	fair	some
7	F.B.	M	fair	some
8	F.B.	F	poor	some
9	F.B.	M	poor	a lot
10	F.B.	F	fair	some
11	F.B.	F	fair	some
12	F.B.	M	very good	all the time
13	F.B.	F	good	all the time
14	F.B.	F	very good	some
15	L.H.	M	poor	some
16	L.H.	M	good	all the time
17	L.H.	F	good	all the time
18	L.H.	M	poor	all the time
19	L.H.	M	poor	all the time
20	L.H.	M	poor	all the time
21	L.H.	M	poor	all the time
22	L.H.	F	excellent	all the time
23	L.H.	F	none	all the time
24	L.H.	F	poor	some
25	L.H.	F	fair	some
26	L.H.	M	poor	all the time
27	L.H.	M	poor	some
28	L.H.	M	good	all the time

Table 1 (Continued)

Respondent	Village	Sex	Signing Ability (self reported)	Contact with Deaf People
29	O.T.	M	none	a little
30	O.T.	F	very good	a lot
31	O.T.	F	none	none
32	O.T.	F	good	some
33	O.T.	F	none	none
34	O.T.	F	none	some
35	O.T.	M	poor	some
36	O.T.	M	fair	some
37	O.T.	M	fair	some
38	O.T.	F	fair	all the time
39	O.T.	F	good	all the time
40	O.T.	M	none	some
41	O.T.	F	poor	a little
42	O.T.	F	good	some
43	M.	F	good	some
44	M.	F	fair	some
45	M.	F	poor	some
46	M.	M	none	none
47	M.	F	none	none
48	M.	F	none	none
49	M.	M	good	some
50	R.P.	F	fair	some
51	R.P.	F	fair	all the time
52	R.P.	F	very good	some
53	R.P.	M	none	none
54	R.P.	F	good	all the time
55	R.P.	M	good	all the time
56	R.P.	M	very good	all the time
57	R.P.	F	good	a lot

responses of an equal number of males and females, however, present working conditions precluded this. As expected, there is more reported contact with Deaf individuals in villages where there are Deaf adults who prefer signing. Also, with the exception of F.B., reported signing ability is generally higher where Deaf adults reside and prefer signing.

Each of the respondents were visited in their own houses. The investigators indicated their desire to know how Hearing people felt about Deaf people and about sign language on the island. During the course of conversations on these topics, nine questions were asked regarding Deaf people and seven questions were asked regarding Providence Island Sign Language. Interviews were conducted in F.B. and L.H. in 1977 by two people from the United States. Later, to check for possible interviewer biases, interviews in O.T. were conducted by the same two researchers and an islander. Furthermore, the interviews in M. and R.P. were completed by the island researcher in the absence of two researchers from the United States.

The questions are presented and discussed below. One word of caution is in order. Providence Islanders use an English creole, and in the questions the term "dumb" as used there means 'profoundly deaf from birth or an early age,' the term "half-dumb" means 'hard of hearing from birth or an early age.' The term "deaf" in the islanders' usage means 'deaf or hard of hearing because of old age.' Expressions with the term "dumb" on Providence do not carry any negative connotations of muteness or stupidity, as they do in U.S. usage. In fact it is common to hear expressions like "X is dumb, but (s)he is very intelligent;" or "X is dumb, but (s)he can say some words." In translating our questions from Providence creole into American English for this paper, we have kept the term "dumb"; obviously it must be interpreted in the context of Providence Island usage.

Deaf People on Providence Island

Marriage

Traditional doctrine in U.S. education for the deaf has held that if deaf people are to marry, they should only marry Hearing people, either to reduce the possibility of deaf children, or to eliminate the "clannishness" Deaf people are supposed to exhibit. This attitude is as old as formal education of the Deaf in the U.S.; e.g. thus, Edward Miner Gallaudet, a Hearing educator of the deaf and first president of the college that bears his name states:

> And even these alumni meetings (of the deaf) will not be without their evils, since by bringing the sexes together they induce intermarriage among deaf-mutes, which we are constrained to deprecate *in toto*, while we would permit the deaf to marry hearing persons with no other let or hinderance (sic) than those existing in the community at large (1873: 202).

And also,

> Everything that serves to draw class lines about them, to intensify their feelings that they are members of a society with interests apart from the mass, to foster the idea that even after leaving school they still, though scattered in widely-separated places, form a "commu-

nity", with leaders and rulers, its associations and organs, and its channels of communication (cf Stokoe, Bernard, and Padden 1976), does undoubtedly tend to make them deafer and more dumb (ibid., 201).

Actually, such negative attitudes have done very little to affect marriage patterns among Deaf people. Fay (1898) records an 85% rate of endogamous marriage among the deaf; and Rainer et al. (1963), in a survey of the deaf in New York, found that 95% of marriages of women born deaf and 91% of women who became deaf at an early age were endogamous.

In order to compare attitudes on marriage cross-culturally, our study posed three questions related to the marriage of Deaf people on Providence: (1) Do you think dumb people should get married? (2) Do you think they should marry people that can hear, other dumb people, or it doesn't matter? (3) Who do you think will have more dumb children: dumb people or people that can hear? Table 2 shows the responses to these questions.

The majority of respondents said that Deaf people should get married if they wanted; this despite the fact that none of the eleven Deaf people of marriageable age on Providence are married. (Not included are one person hard of hearing and those born on Providence who have moved away and not kept close contact—note that with a population of 3,000, the island might be expected to have between 3 and 6 deaf persons.) In Providence Island as in the U.S., there is a strong tendency for respondents to advocate marriage of the Deaf with Hearing persons; but the reasons given differ: The respondents on Providence do not cite reasons like those of E.M. Gallaudet but say that having a Hearing partner might help the Deaf person in a fire or a burglary or other emergency where they believe Hearing is crucial. It should be pointed out that almost half of the Deaf adults have children even though they are not married—it is common on Providence for both married and unmarried persons (Hearing and Deaf) to have children. Having children out of wedlock does not carry as much prestige but it still brings much positive "reputation" to the biological parents. (See Wilson, 1973, for a discussion of reputation.)

As question (3) indicates people on Providence generally know that the deaf children on Providence have hearing parents. Although almost half the Deaf people on Providence have had children, they have had only hearing children.

Abilities of Deaf People

Because Deaf people have traditionally been considered pathologically handicapped individuals in the U.S. rather than members of a minority group (Padden & Markowicz 1976, Markowicz & Woodward 1975), it is not surprising to find in this country negative attitudes about the intelligence,

TABLE 2

Responses of Providence Islanders to marriage questions.

Question	Response	Evaluation	In F.B. No.	%	In L.H. No.	%	In O.T. No.	%	In M. No.	%	In R.P. No.	%	Total No.	%
1. Do you think dumb people should get married?	yes	+	9	64	11	79	14	100	6	86	7	88	47	82
	no	−	5	36	3	21	0	0	1	14	1	13	10	18
2. Do you think they should marry people that can hear, other dumb people, or it doesn't matter?	dumb people	+	2	14	3	21	3	21	0	0	1	13	9	16
	doesn't matter	+	2	14	1	7	2	14	0	0	0	0	5	9
	people that can hear	−	5	36	7	50	9	64	6	86	6	75	33	58
	predicted by q. 1	−	5	36	3	21	0	0	1	14	1	13	10	18
3. Who do you think will have more dumb children: dumb people or people that can hear?	doesn't matter	+	0	0	0	0	1	7	2	29	0	0	3	5
	people that can hear	+	9	64	12	86	9	64	4	57	6	75	40	70
	dumb people	−	5	36	1	7	2	14	1	14	1	13	10	18
	don't know		0	0	1	7	2	14	0	0	1	13	4	7

maturity, and mental health of Deaf people. Mindel and Vernon (1971) summarized 38 major studies of the intelligence of deaf and hard of hearing individuals in a 37-year span between 1930 and 1967 and concluded that it is not uncommon to find people equating speech in a deaf person with intelligence, nor is it uncommon to find a deaf person with easily intelligible speech rated far superior in intelligence to a deaf person with difficult to understand speech, despite an opposite difference in actual mental ability.

Immaturity also has its stereotypes. Deaf individuals in traditional studies are often called immature, impulsive, or tactless; but these judgements are often from the Hearing society's point of view. It is just as common to find personality stereotypes for other minority groups; e.g. these: "Blacks are not intellectual, but they make good athletes;" and "Spanish people are so happy; they sing and dance all day." But it should be remembered that acceptable personality traits vary from culture to culture. Furth, a psychologist familiar with the Deaf, puts it well:

> Thus the personality of a person cannot be separated from the social world in which he functions. An apparently introverted deaf child in the hearing world can become an extrovert in the deaf society, and an immature, unsuccessful schoolboy can become an adult who leads a mature, constructive life in his community (Furth 1973: 83).

Hearing individuals and institutions in the U.S. have been known to confuse deafness with mental disease. One hears stories of deaf people being locked up in mental institutions for years before being released because by chance someone tested their hearing and found that they were only deaf. The prevalence of such stories may suggest that this situation cannot exist now, but it does. I have just become aware that a student now at Gallaudet College had been placed in a mental institution and remained there for several years before she was found to be merely hard of hearing. She is still taking medication to counteract the adverse physical effects of the drugs administered for the mental illness she never had in the first place!

Another situation, not so drastic but equally depressing, is one that Furth points out:

> Teachers and counselors in a residential school for deaf children rated 11.5% of the children as severely disturbed and 19.5% as moderately disturbed, compared to 2.5% and 7.5% for an entire public school system. One suspects that the ratings for the deaf children encompass an emotionally unhealthy atmosphere in which parents, teachers, and counselors, and the entire school system are involved (Furth 1973: 81).

Our study asked three questions related to the abilities of Deaf people, specifically related to intelligence, maturity, and mental health: (4) Imagine you compare dumb people and people that can hear. Are dumb people more smart, the same smart, or less smart than people that can hear? (5) Are dumb people as mature as people that can hear? Can they take the same responsibilities as people that can hear? (6) Are the dumb people more probable, the same probable, or less probable to have problems with nerves? Table 3 shows the responses to these questions. These responses indicate positive attitudes on the part of the great majority of respondents about the intelligence, maturity, and mental health of Deaf people on Providence.

There were two differences in responses that should be commented on. First, relating to the intelligence of Deaf people, a number of respondents in O.T. and R.P. indicated that Deaf people had the ability to be as intelligent as Hearing people, but that they needed training if they were to achieve that intelligence. In other words, intelligence for these people is something that must be cultivated. This response did not appear in the F.B., L.H., or on M.

Second, relating to question 5, the majority of people in M. indicated that Deaf people were not always able to look out for themselves. The reason given for this response by the Hearing people was that not all Hearing people could understand signs on Providence. Therefore, the Deaf people might need the help of a Hearing interpreter in these situations. While we have included this as a negative response in comparison with the response of other islanders, we feel that the response indicates a lack of abilities of Hearing people rather than a lack of abilities of Deaf people. Also this response does not necessarily indicate an attitude toward maturity per se. It certainly is much less severe than the type of attitude toward Deaf people in the United States discussed by Woodward (1975) and Furth (1973).

Occupational Equality

In most of the industrial world, there has been a great deal of discrimination against Deaf people in the areas of social and economic equality. As Furth points out:

> . . .deafness used to be a legal obstacle to getting a driver's license in many states and countries, although a deaf person can obtain a license in all the United States and Canada. However, insurance is a major problem. What about their driving record? Does not a lack of hearing contribute to a greater accident rate? The facts show that deaf drivers have a better record than others (1973: 4).

Nowhere, however, has discrimination been more severe than in jobs and pay. Schein and Delk state:

> A number of studies have found employers reluctant to hire deaf workers (Rickard, Triandis, & Patterson 1963, Williams 1972). Rickard

TABLE 3

Responses to questions on the abilities of Deaf people.

Question	Response	Evaluation	In F.B. No.	%	In L.H. No.	%	In O.T. No.	%	In M. No.	%	In R.P. No.	%	Total No.	%
4. Are dumb people more smart, the same smart, or less smart than people that can hear?	more smart	+	0	0	5	36	3	21	4	57	1	13	13	23
	same smart	+	9	64	4	29	3	21	2	29	0	0	18	32
	same (with training)	+	0	0	0	0	4	29	0	0	6	75	10	18
	m. or s. (depends)	+	0	0	2	14	0	0	0	0	0	0	2	4
	less smart	–	5	36	3	21	4	29	1	14	0	0	13	23
	don't know		0	0	0	0	0	0	0	0	1	13	1	2
5. Are dumb people as mature. . . ? Can they take the same responsibilities . . ? (Can they look for themselves?)	yes	+	12	86	11	79	12	86	3	43	8	100	46	81
	no	–	2	14	3	21	2	14	4	57	0	0	11	19
6. Are dumb people more probable, same probable, or less probable to have problems with nerves?	same probable	+	5	36	6	43	10	71	2	29	5	63	28	49
	less probable	+	6	43	8	57	1	7	3	43	2	25	20	35
	more probable	–	1	7	0	0	2	14	2	29	1	13	6	11
	don't know		2	14	0	0	1	7	0	0	0	0	3	5

et al. found general prejudice against hiring disabled applicants. Deafness was rated worse than tuberculosis and wheelchair-bound and better than epilepsy, ex-prison, and ex-mental hospital by personnel directors. Similar ratings were given by school administrators, except when the hypothetical applicant sought a position as a third-grade teacher. Then the deaf applicant rated worse than all but the epileptic (1974: 89).

Regarding pay, the same authors find:

> The deaf individuals' median incomes are from 62 to 76 percent of their general population peers. Overall deaf earnings are 72 percent of those for individuals at large. White deaf females do best, earning 76 percent as much as white females. The remaining contrasts with their general counterparts show nonwhite deaf males at 62 percent, white deaf males 74 percent, and nonwhite deaf females 62 percent of corresponding earnings (Schein & Delk 1974: 101).

However, it should be remembered that the above statistics are for "prevocationally" deaf people, i.e. people who became deaf up to the age of nineteen. Many of these people are thus not core members of the U.S. Deaf community. In the United States,

> personal earnings are directly related to age at onset of deafness. Those born deaf have the lowest average, and those who lost their hearing after age 7, the highest. The difference between the medium is $1,208, a substantial sum (Schein & Delk 1974: 103).

Our study asked two questions related to the occupational equality of Deaf people: (7) Can dumb people get the same jobs as people that can hear? (8) When dumb people have the same job as a person that can hear, do they get the same pay? Table 4 shows the responses.

The responses to these questions about occupations are extremely interesting. The large number of negative responses to question 7 indicates the changing of a self-sufficient economy on Providence Island to a cash economy with the resulting specialization of labor. All respondents who indicated that Deaf people could not get the same jobs as Hearing people also indicated that the type of jobs Deaf people could not get involved office work that demanded contact with people from all over the island; e.g. jobs in the bank or post office. It was felt this work would be difficult for the Deaf to get, since depending on the location of their village, Hearing people may or may not be fluent in signs. In addition, signs vary considerably from region to region in this small island. (It is ironic that in the highly specialized U.S. economy, the Post Office is one place where Deaf people easily find jobs, as sorters; Providence is not large enough to need even one sorter.)

TABLE 4

Responses to questions on occupational equality of Deaf people.

Question	Response	Evaluation	In F.B. No.	%	In L.H. No.	%	In O.T. No.	%	In M. No.	%	In R.P. No.	%	Total No.	%
7. Can dumb people get the same jobs as people that can hear?	yes	+	6	43	3	21	5	36	3	43	4	50	21	37
	no	–	8	57	11	79	9	64	4	57	4	50	36	63
8. When dumb people have the same job as a person that can hear, do they get the same pay?	yes	+	12	86	14	100	14	100	6	86	8	100	54	95
	no	–	2	14	0	0	0	0	1	14	0	0	3	5

From the responses to question 7, it would appear that Deaf people are primarily socialized into their immediate communities rather than into the whole island economy. Unfortunately, if the trend toward specialization continues, Deaf people may slowly become more isolated from the mainstream community.

Question 8 indicates, however, that the majority of respondents still feel that Deaf people get the same pay for their work as do Hearing people. By carefully questioning people other than respondents about appropriate pay for Deaf consultants and Deaf workers, we have seen that Deaf people do in fact make the same wages as Hearing people on the same jobs, and are expected to.

Social Integration

Deaf people in the United States are often not assimilated into the majority Hearing culture. Some Hearing educators (e.g. Gallaudet in the work cited) have commented on the "clannishness" of Deaf people, but the majority view in the Hearing world is that Deaf people are isolated pathological individuals. Contrary to both of these views, Deaf people in the U.S. form a thriving community, one held together by such factors as self-identification as a member of a Deaf community (Padden & Markowicz 1976, Markowicz & Woodward 1975), endogamous marital patterns (Fay 1898, Rainer et al. 1963), and numerous national, regional, and local organizations and social structures (Meadow 1972)—even an elite, power controlling structure (Stokoe, Bernard, & Padden 1976). Not all hearing-impaired individuals belong to the Deaf community. In fact, audiometric deafness, the measured degree of hearing loss, often has very little to do with where a person fits in the Deaf community (Padden & Markowicz 1976). Attitudinal Deafness (self-identification as a member of the Deaf community plus identification by other members as one of them) appears to be the most powerful factor determining membership. Attitudinal Deafness also explains why some hard of hearing persons consider themselves Deaf, why some with profound loss claim to be hard of hearing or able to hear, and why some young children of Deaf parents may refuse to speak for some time, even though they are quite capable of hearing and speaking.

The situation on Providence Island is very different. Deaf people on Providence do not form a community, but in fact are fairly well integrated into the daily activities of the island (see Washabaugh, Woodward, De Santis 1978). In our interviews we asked this final question: (9) Do dumb people go around and talk with everyone on the island or do they keep to themselves? All the respondents from L.H., M., R.P., and all but one of the respondents from F.B. and two from O.T. indicated that Deaf individuals are not isolated but indeed do associate with everyone and talk with everyone just as Hearing people do (talk in this case refers to the islanders' sign language of course).

Sign Language on Providence Island

The Origin of Sign Language

Studies of sign language and the education of the deaf in the United States often remark upon the fact that T.H. Gallaudet and L. Clerc brought French Sign Language to the U.S. This seems a very unsatisfactory explanation from what is known about language variation and change. Gallaudet was a Hearing American with minimal training in French Sign Language. Clerc was a French deaf man who apparently advocated assimilation into the Hearing community. It is also a little ethnocentric to assume that Deaf people in the U.S. could not have developed their own sign language as the Deaf people on Providence have. In histories of the education of the deaf in the U.S., Gallaudet gets the lion's share of the credit, while Clerc plays the role of a helper.

Woodward (1978) has hypothesized that there were sign languages in use in the U.S. before 1816, that is, before French Sign Language was brought to the U.S. It appears that French Sign Language was creolized with existing varieties of sign language in the U.S. producing modern American Sign Language. Glottochronological procedures show extremely large lexical differences between modern French Sign Language and modern American Sign Language, even though they have been separated for only 160 years. The existence of indigenous sign varieties in the U.S. would explain this discrepancy.

In order to compare the beliefs on the origins of sign language crossculturally and thus to compare attitudes about the ability of Deaf people to create their own language, our study posed two questions related to the origins of Providence Island Sign Language: (1) Did the dumb people's signs come from Providence or did someone bring them from some other place? (2) Who do you think first made the signs on Providence: the hearing people, the dumb people, or the dumb and hearing people together? Table 5 shows the response to these questions.

Only one person (2% of the sample) said that someone brought the signs to Providence. Six people (11% of the sample) stated that Hearing people alone were responsible for inventing Providence Island Sign Language.

Universality or Uniqueness of Sign Language

Belief that sign language is universal is very widespread. Battison and Jordan (1976: 54) point out a number of well know works on sign language that express this belief. This belief indicates that sign language is basically

TABLE 5

Responses of Providence Islanders to questions about the origins of Providence Island Sign Language.

Question	Response	Evaluation	In F.B. No.	%	In L.H. No.	%	In O.T. No.	&	In M. No.	%	In R.P. No.	%	Total No.	%
1. Did the dumb people's signs come from Providence or did someone bring them from some other place?	From Providence	+	13	93	14	100	12	86	4	57	8	100	51	89
	From another place	–	0	0	0	0	0	0	1	14	0	0	1	2
	Don't know		1	7	0	0	2	14	2	29	0	0	5	9
2. Who do you think first made the signs on Providence: the hearing people, the dumb people, or the dumb and hearing people together?	Dumb people	+	9	64	12	86	9	64	3	43	6	75	39	68
	Dumb and hearing people	+	0	0	0	0	0	0	3	43	1	13	4	7
	Hearing people	–	3	21	1	7	1	7	1	14	0	0	6	11
	Don't know		2	14	1	7	4	29	0	0	1	13	8	14

different from oral language in that it does not vary and tends to imply that sign language does not have to be learned or at least it can be learned with no problem because it is somehow easier or simpler than oral languages. According to Battison and Jordan (1976: 61–62):

> Some signers in America tend to think of all European sign languages as being vaguely the same entity and are often surprised at the complexity and differences among European sign languages. We have two illustrations of this contrast: (a) In the course of introducing a Dane to some Americans, the Canadian introducer used a few Danish signs. One of the Americans remarked to him, "Oh, you know International Sign Language!" (b) A European teacher of the deaf who is deaf himself, spent a year as a graduate student at Gallaudet. An American student asked him if he planned to take American Sign Language back to his country. The teacher looked surprised and said, "No, what for? We have our own sign language in my country." The student was astonished. Prior to his departure for the U.S., the same teacher had announced to his class of ten-year-old deaf pupils that he was going to America for a year of study. The class erupted with expressions of dismay. When asked why they thought it was so terrible, the pupils answered, "Because you'll have to learn American Sign Language!" These European youngsters who had seen many foreign deaf people come and go, had a clear idea of the separation of different sign languages; while the older American college students did not.

In order to compare beliefs on the universality of sign language, our study posed the following question: (3) Do dumb people all around the world sign the same so they can understand each other or do dumb people have to learn each other's signs if they go to another place? Table 6 shows the responses.

The responses across all villages are very consistent. The majority of respondents said that sign language was not universal but had to be learned. In addition, most of these respondents also pointed out that there was even regional variation in Providence Island Sign Language. Only 14% of the people interviewed believed that sign language was universal. There is an obvious difference in the beliefs and resultant attitudes of Providence Islanders and those of specialists and lay people in the U.S.

The Grammar of Sign Language

Linguists who study American Sign Language have frequently remarked that the mainstream attitude in both Hearing and Deaf communities has been that American Sign Language has no grammar or is poor or broken language (Stokoe 1970, Markowicz 1972, among others). Battison and Jordan (1976: 53) point out the problem quite well:

TABLE 6

Responses of Providence Islanders to the question about universality of sign language.

Question	Response	Evaluation	In F.B. No.	%	In L.H. No.	%	In O.T. No.	%	In M. No.	%	In R.P. No.	%	Total No.	%
3. Do dumb people all around the world sign the same so that they can understand each other or do the dumb people have to learn each other's signs if they go to another place?	different—learn new signs	+	11	79	12	86	11	79	6	86	7	88	47	82
	can understand each other (universal)	−	3	21	2	14	2	14	1	14	0	0	8	14
	don't know		0	0	0	0	1	7	0	0	1	13	2	4

Others believe that sign languages have no grammar, no "proper" ways of expressing things, but merely "throw together" gestures and pantomimic actions; or they believe that sign languages abridge and corrupt correct spoken language grammar. These myths have been treated in recent years by other researchers, who find that the formal structures and communicative functions of sign languages used by deaf people are comparable to those of spoken languages used by hearing people (Stokoe 1960, 1970, Woodward 1973; Battison 1974; Bellugi & Klima 1975; Baker 1975; Frishberg 1975; Klima & Bellugi 1975; Liddell 1975; Padden & Markowicz 1975; Stokoe & Battison 1975).

Empirical research usually has little effect on attitudes, however. Witness the following classical attitudes from George Johnston, "Who has been deaf since the age of five and is presently (as of 1977) only a dissertation short of a doctorate in special education administration, (and who) is director of Project PALS a federally-funded statewide project designed to provide alternate language skills for Deaf students" (Marose 1977).

What Belugi (sic) in California and other people are calling American Sign Language or Ameslan, or as lazy and brief as they like to get, ASL, is actually Deaf English. DEAF ENGLISH is the typical errors (from improper or insufficient exposure) to English. It is a choice of words, a sub-culture style, omissions and additions, etc. . .

Give an English paragraph to 100 deaf people and ask them to sign it in American Sign Language. You will find them all different—no syntax. Only some common habits will be noticed.

Then I argue, "What is syntax? How can you call American Sign Language something with a syntax when syntax involves sentence structure. Ridiculous, it is just Broken English or DEAF ENGLISH (Johnston 1977: 22).

Our study asked two questions related to the grammar of sign language: (4) Is there a proper order for signs? and (5) Do you think the signs are a different language from the patois (Providence Island creole)? Table 7 shows the responses from the five villages. The majority of the respondents indicated that there is a proper order for signs and that the sign language is a different language from the spoken language. This is in contrast to the traditional attitudes in the educational establishment for the Deaf in the U.S.

The Effectiveness of Communication in Sign Language

As Markowicz (1972: 27) points out: even "when it is accepted as a system of communication, sign language is often not considered equal to other natural languages."

TABLE 7

Responses of Providence Islanders to questions about the grammar of sign language.

Question	Response	Evaluation	In F.B. No.	%	In L.H. No.	%	In O.T. No.	%	In M. No.	%	In R.P. No.	%	Total No.	%
4. Is there a proper order for the signs?	yes	+	9	64	10	71	13	93	4	57	8	100	44	77
	no	–	4	29	4	29	1	7	3	43	0	0	12	21
	don't know		1	7	0	0	0	0	0	0	0	0	1	2
5. Do you think the signs are a different language from the patois?	yes	+	8	57	8	57	7	50	5	71	8	100	36	63
	no	–	5	36	5	36	5	36	2	29	0	0	17	30
	don't know		1	7	1	7	2	14	0	0	0	0	4	7

Tervoort claims "that the material he recorded on film for his study on young deaf children contained very few instances of metaphoric, ironic, or humorous usages." (Markowicz 1972: 28). On the other hand, Klima and Bellugi (1975) report a wealth of humorous and poetic capability in American Sign Language.

Our study posed the following question in relation to the effectiveness of communication of Providence Island Sign Language: (6) Can dumb people express everything they want to say in the signs or are they limited? Table 8 shows the responses to this question.

The majority of respondents (68%) said that Deaf people on Providence could express everything they wanted to say in Providence Island Sign Language. With the exception of those who live in M., the majority of respondents in each village expressed this positive attitude. It should be remembered that the deaf people in M. are young and do not prefer to use signs. Thus the difference of attitude in M. is easily explainable.

The Rights of Deaf People to Use Sign Language

Sign language usage in the U.S. has flourished despite subtle and sometimes not so subtle pressures. The major issue in language policy for deaf education has been the oral-manual controversy. Oralism has been advocated strongly since the 1880 International Conference of Teachers of the Deaf met in Milan and declared: "The Congress, considering the incontestable superiority of speech over signing in restoring the deaf mute to society, and in giving him a more perfect knowledge of language, declares that the oral method ought to be preferred to that of signs for the education of the deaf and dumb."

It should be pointed out that even the advocates of manualism are not generally purely manual but often advocate a combined method of speech and signs that parallel English word order.

As a result of educational policy, audiologists and doctors, two groups whom Hearing parents often rely on for information on deaf children, also advocate oralism, usually with the argument that signing will impede speech and language development (naturally this assumes that ASL is not a language). What is particularly interesting, however, is that as Markowicz (1972: 24) points out:

". . . several extensive research studies (Meadow 1967, Montgomery 1966, Stevenson 1964, Quigley and Frisina 1961, Quigley 1969, Stuckless and Birch 1966, Vernon 1969) have shown that children with early manual communication not only are more advanced when they enter school, but maintain this advantage throughout their school age years." (Campbell 1970: 15) The results of these studies indicate that in a comparison of them with children who have been brought up orally

TABLE 8

Responses of Providence Islanders to questions about effectiveness of communication in Providence Island Sign Language.

Question	Response	Evaluation	In F.B.		In L.H.		In O.T.		In M.		In R.P.		Total	
			No.	%	No.	%	No.	%	No.	%	No.	%	No.	%
6. Can dumb people express everything they want to say in the signs or are they limited?	Can express	+	8	57	8	57	13	93	2	29	8	100	39	68
	Limited	−	6	43	6	43	1	7	5	71	0	0	18	32

only, the former generally have a better command of language, not only in manual communication, but also in lipreading, reading and writing. There was no difference in speech intelligibility between the two groups.

Our study asked the following question related to the rights of Deaf people to use sign language: (7) Do you think the dumb people ought to learn to talk, the hearing people ought to learn to sign like the dumb people, or that both the dumb people and hearing people ought to learn the other's way of communication? Table 9 shows the responses to this question.

The majority of respondents from all villages said that Hearing people should learn to sign. Only 11% of the respondents said that Deaf people should learn to talk and Hearing people need not learn to sign.

Summary and Conclusions

The research in this paper, conducted in five villages, has supported field observations of relatively positive attitudes toward Deaf people and toward sign language held by Hearing people on Providence Island. From comparisons with traditional attitudes toward Deaf people and toward sign language in educational institutions in the United States, it appears that Providence Island indeed has a more positive attitude toward Deaf people and sign language.

While Deaf people on Providence have not married, there is no stigma attached to having children out of wedlock; professed attitudes are at least as positive as in the United States. 70% of the respondents believe (correctly) that the union of two hearing people is more likely to cause deafness on Providence than the union of a deaf person with a hearing person or other deaf person. Engagements in the United States have been broken up by doctors' suggestions that a mixed (hearing and deaf) couple might have even a slight possibility of having deaf children.

Deaf people are viewed as equally intelligent or more intelligent (77%), equally mature (81%), and less likely to have mental problems (35%) or at least no more likely to have mental problems (an additional 49%) as compared with Hearing people. In contrast, the educational establishment in the United States has been extremely concerned with all of these areas, frequently approaching overkill in testing and labelling Deaf individuals as inferior.

Finally, while the introduction of a cash economy on Providence Island is creating specialization of jobs and resulting in some discrimination against Deaf people, now at least Deaf people still receive the same pay as Hearing. As we have pointed out, the employment and compensation situation in the United States is quite discriminatory against the average Deaf person.

TABLE 9

Responses of Providence Islanders to the question about the rights of Deaf people to use sign language.

Question	Response	Evaluation	In F.B. No.	%	In L.H. No.	%	In O.T. No.	%	In M. No.	%	In R.P. No.	%	Total No.	%
7. Do you think the dumb people ought to learn to talk, the hearing people ought to learn to sign like the dumb people, or that both the dumb people and hearing people ought to learn each other's way of communicating?	hearing sign	+	8	57	9	64	14	100	6	86	8	100	45	79
	hearing sign and dumb talk	+	2	14	3	21	0	0	0	0	0	0	5	9
	dumb talk	–	4	29	1	7	0	0	1	14	0	0	6	11
	don't know		0	0	1	7	0	0	0	0	0	0	1	2

In relation to Providence Island Sign Language, only one (2%) of the respondents indicated that they believed that Providence Island Sign Language did not develop indigenously, 11% gave sole credit to Hearing people (parents) for the development of Providence Island Sign Language. Only 14% believed that sign language is universal. The majority of respondents believed that Providence Island Sign Language had a grammar (77%), and was a different language from the spoken language (63%). The majority of respondents also indicated that Deaf people could express anything they wished in Providence Island Sign Language (68%). Most importantly over three-fourths of the respondents (79%) stated that the Hearing people should learn signs rather than Deaf people having to learn to talk, while only 11% of the respondents indicated that the Deaf people should learn to talk without it being necessary for Hearing people to sign.

We feel these findings can be generalized to the population of Providence Island, since we have surveyed representatives from about two-thirds of the area and over 40% of the population (see Wilson, 1973). The findings are strengthened further since respondents in the last two villages were interviewed by a different investigator, who is also a member of the society.

References

Battison, R. and I.K. Jordan. 1976. Cross Cultural Communication with Foreign Signers: Fact and Fancy. *Sign Language Studies* 10, 53–68.

Fay, E.A. 1898. *Marriages of the Deaf in America.* Washington, D.C.: The Volta Bureau.

Furth, H. 1973. *Deafness and Learning: A Psychological Approach.* Belmont, CA: Wadsworth.

Gallaudet, E.M. 1873. "Deaf-Mute" Conventions, Associations, and Newspapers. *American Annals of the Deaf* 18:2, 200–206.

Johnston, G. 1977. George's Scope: The Confusing Terminology: Crisis for 1977, 1978, 1979, etc. *The Deaf Spectrum*, 20–25.

Klima, E. and U. Bellugi. 1975. Wit and Poetry in American Sign Language. *Sign Language Studies* 8, 203–224.

Markowicz, H. 1972. Some Sociolinguistic Considerations of American Sign Language. *Sign Language Studies* 1, 15–41.

Markowicz, H. and J. Woodward. 1975 (1978, 1982). Language and the Maintenance of Ethnic Boundaries in the Deaf Community. Paper presented at the Conference on Culture & Communication. Philadelphia. Published in *Communication and Cognition* Vol. 11, No. 1 and in this volume.

Marose, S. 1972. Sign Language Aids Deaf Kids to Speak. *The Deaf Spectrum* 1–2.

Meadow, K. 1972. Sociolinguistics, Sign Language, and the Deaf Subculture. In T.J. O'Rourke ed. *Psycholinguistics and Total Communication: The State of the Art*, 1–10. Silver Spring, MD: American Annals of the Deaf.

Mindel, E. and M. Vernon. 1971. *They Grow in Silence.* Silver Spring, MD: National Association of the Deaf.

Padden, C. and H. Markowicz. 1976. Cultural Conflicts between Hearing and Deaf Communities. In Crammatte and Crammatte, eds. *VII World Congress of the Deaf*, 407–411. Silver Spring, MD: National Association of the Deaf.

Rainer, J.D., K.Z. Altshuler, and F.J. Kallman, eds. 1963. *Family and Mental Health Problems in a Deaf Population*. New York: State Psychiatric Institute, Columbia.

Rickard, T.E., E.C. Triandis, and C.H. Patterson. 1963. Indices of Employer Prejudice Toward Disabled Applicants, *Journal of Applied Psychology* 47, 52–55.

Schein, J.D. and M. Delk. 1974. *The Deaf Population of the United States*. Silver Spring, MD: National Association of the Deaf.

Stokoe, W. 1970. Sign Language Diglossia. *Studies in Linguistics* 21, 27–41.

Stokoe, W., H. Bernard, and C. Padden. 1976. An Elite Group in Deaf Society. *Sign Language Studies* 12, 189–210.

Washabaugh, W., J. Woodward, and S. De Santis. 1978. Providence Island Sign Language: A Context-Dependent Language. *Anthropological Linguistics* (March), 95–109.

Williams, C.A. 1972. Is Hiring the Handicapped Good Business? *Journal of Rehabilitation* (March/April), 30–34.

Wilson, P. 1973. *Crab Antics*. New Haven: Yale Univ. Press.

Woodward J. 1975 (1982). How You Gonna Get to Heaven if You Can't Talk With Jesus: The Educational Establishment vs. The Deaf Community. Paper presented at the Society for Applied Anthropology, Amsterdam. Published in this volume.

Woodward, J. 1978. Historical Bases of American Sign Language. In P. Siple, ed. *Understanding Language Through Sign Language Research*, 333–348. New York: Academic Press.

James Woodward

On Depathologizing Deafness

The papers in this book have demonstrated that there are two opposing views of Deaf people and their relationship to the larger U.S. society. These different views are part of two different cultural value systems: Hearing ideology and Deaf ideology. We have attempted in the papers to describe Deaf people in a way that is consistent with their own ideology and that is consistent with accurate and currently accepted anthropological and sociolinguistic measures.

The Hearing ideological perspective that Deaf people who identify with the Deaf community are isolated pathological handicapped individuals is not borne out by careful scientific anthropological and linguistic analyses. Yet the fact remains that Hearing people are slow and many times reluctant to relinquish their cultural values concerning Deaf people, even though they may be harmful and repressive to Deaf people.

Thus certain basic cultural values in Deaf and Hearing societies are in conflict, since they are based on opposing views of the nature of Deaf people. Power, money, upward social mobility, etc. in U.S. society are basically controlled by those in authority, namely the Hearing majority culture. This results in inequalities in regard to Deaf people, since access to social and economic success is controlled by a culture with an ideology that tends to consider Deaf people as inferior.

One cannot deny that over the last few years there has been some improvement in attitudes towards Deaf people and American Sign Language and that there have been some economic benefits to Deaf people, but Deaf people are still far from being equal to Hearing people in U.S. society. One only has to examine the legislation affecting the rights of Deaf people to see that Deaf people are still classified as handicapped. Deaf people are almost never classified with other minority groups. It is very improbable that Deaf people will ever achieve equality, unless Hearing society depathologizes deafness: that is, unless Hearing society rejects the handicapped classification of Deaf people.

For if we look more closely at the notion of "handicapped" and its ramifications, we come to a rather unpleasant logical conclusion. *The American Heritage Dictionary* (1976) defines 'handicap' as a "deficiency, especially an anatomical, physiological, or mental deficiency, that prevents or restricts normal achievement." If we follow the traditional handicapped classification of Deaf people, Deaf people are doomed to failure because they will never achieve (nor do they always want to "achieve") the "normality" of becoming a Hearing person. Most Deaf people will then remain (according to Hearing society's norms) "deficient," that is "lacking an essential quality or element; incomplete; defective." (The American Heritage Dictionary, 1976).

The handicapped classification of Deaf people is detrimental to Deaf people. The most serious detriment to Deaf people is the fact that to be classified as handicapped means to be given the label of inferior. It really matters little in the long run how much temporary money we provide for services for Deaf people, if we still classify them as second class citizens with the label of handicapped. The money will not last forever, or possibly for very long. And when the money is gone, the inferior social label will assure that Deaf people once again are definitely placed in their "appropriate" inferior place (Woodward 1980). Value change must accompany the economic benefits if permanent social benefit is to accrue to Deaf people.

In addition to being detrimental to Deaf people, the handicapped classification of Deaf people is also detrimental to Hearing people. The detriment to Hearing people is more subtle, yet perhaps more serious. By labelling Deaf people as handicapped, we reject Deaf culture, Deaf values, and the self-worth of Deaf people. By saying Deaf are handicapped we are saying they really are inferior. By using the term handicapped, we have placed ourselves, consciously or unconsciously, in the role of oppressor. We have said Deaf people have a "deficiency, especially an anatomical, physiological, or mental deficiency, that prevents or restricts normal achievement." We have thus made it clear that Deaf people can succeed only if they follow Hearing rules and only to the extent they can become like Hearing people. When we send Deaf children to doctors before we try to find Deaf and Hearing adults for them to communicate with, we have made deafness into a pathology, a sickness, that our science feels it must eradicate.

One only has to look at a community like Providence Island to see how much we have pathologized deafness. Hearing people on Providence Island obviously know that Deaf people cannot hear. However, they tend to classify this as a difference rather than a deficit. They do not view hearing as such an "essential" quality as U.S. society does. Moreover, the attitude studies on Providence Island definitely show that Deaf people are not considered "defective." Deafness tends to be accepted as a fact. There is no attempt to find a medical cure or a technological solution for a person who does not hear. Rather Hearing people on Providence Island seek social ways of relating to Deaf people. Deaf people on Providence do not need to become hearing to succeed. Parents of Deaf children on Providence are not concerned with doctors or with hearing aids or with making their children "normal"; they are concerned with communicating with their children and seeing that the children can communicate with others. Again it should be stressed that the situation on Providence Island is not perfect for Deaf individuals, but the more positive attitudes of Hearing people towards the Deaf certainly help toward integrating Deaf people into the larger society.

If we in the United States are truly to accept and treat Deaf people as equal, we must depathologize deafness. This involves rejecting our culture's medical model of deafness. This model is deeply rooted in American Hearing cultural tradition. Changes in our beliefs will not occur overnight, since pathological views of deafness pervade U.S. Hearing society in many subtle ways that are probably only rarely consciously noticed but that undoubtedly have a profound subconscious affect.

The impetus for attitudinal changes towards Deaf individuals should come from both the Deaf and Hearing communities. As pointed out earlier in this book, meaningful social change for the Deaf community cannot be designed solely by Hearing people. Deaf people who have an intimate knowledge of their own community must be involved in every aspect of language and social planning. The Hearing people to be involved in language and social planning related to the Deaf community must also be very knowledgeable about the Deaf community's language varieties and values.

Anyone interested in attitudinal change must also understand why Hearing people have developed the negative attitudes they have. To obtain this understanding, we need (1) more cross cultural studies of beliefs and attitudes towards Deaf people and towards sign languages and (2) a close examination of our own negative attitudes and how they are supported and reinforced by our social institutions, especially by institutions that we consider sacred in one form or another. Two such institutions are our science and our religion. We have already pointed out some of the characteristics of the scientific medical model of deafness. This model advocates intervention with technological devices such as hearing aids or "cure" through surgical procedures. Mainstream religious tradition in the U.S. shares a similar view of deafness. Passages in the Judeo-Christian Bible referring to deafness and Deaf people view deafness as a pathology, something to be cured, usually by God. Thus the Judeo-Christian biblical tradition supports, reinforces, and gives supernatural justification to the U.S. Hearing pathological view of deafness. Many of our other social institutions also view deafness in a similar way.

Perhaps the most difficult task for U.S. society in a quest to depathologize deafness will be to objectively examine, question, and reject such values in such sensitive areas as those described above. As Hsu, an anthropologist, has so aptly observed: "Many Western and especially American scholars have been too emotionally immersed in the absolute goodness of their own form of society, ethic, thought, and religion that it is hard for them to question them, even in scientific analyses." (Hsu 1972:245). Yet, if we do not question our present values, they will remain the same; and Deaf people will remain unequal in our society which claims to value egalitarianism.

References

Hsu, F. 1972. American Core Value and National Character. In F. Hsu, ed., *Psychological Anthropology*. Cambridge, Mass.: Schenkman Publishing Co., Inc.

Morris, M., ed. 1976. *The American Heritage Dictionary of the English Language*. Boston: Houghton Mifflin Company.

Woodward, J. 1980. Cyclic Politics: Sign Language and Deaf Education. A paper presented in the lecture series on Language and the Politics of Education, State University of New York, Binghamton, March.